I0426562

What You Need To Know About Getting In Shape

Tips and Strategies from Top Trainers

South Peak Press

What You Need To Know About Getting In Shape

ISBN: 1492209295
ISBN-13: 978-1492209294

DEDICATION

This book is dedicated to the talented professionals who took the time to submit content for this project. The high quality instruction and encouragement you have all shared has truly gone above and beyond what I expected when I first set out to publish this book. I am convinced those who study and apply your advice will advance their health and improve their lives. My thanks to all who made this book possible.

Andy Adami

for

SouthPeakPress.com

This book is an educational product that provides general health information. The materials in *What You Need To Know About Getting In Shape: Tips And Strategies From Top Trainers* are provided "as is" and without warranties of any kind either express or implied.

AS AN EXPRESS CONDITION TO USING THE INFORMATION IN THIS BOOK, YOU MUST AGREE TO THE FOLLOWING TERMS. IF YOU DISAGREE WITH ANY OF THESE TERMS, DO NOT USE THE INFORMATION IN THIS BOOK. YOUR PARTICIPATION IN ACTIVITIES MENTIONED IN THIS BOOK MEANS THAT YOU ARE AGREEING TO BE LEGALLY BOUND BY THESE TERMS:

This book's content is not a substitute for direct, personal, professional medical care and diagnosis. None of the advice, diet plans, or exercises mentioned should be performed or otherwise used without clearance from your physician or health care provider. The information contained within is not intended to provide specific physical or mental health advice, or any other advice whatsoever, for any individual or company and should not be relied upon in that regard. We are not medical professionals and nothing in this book should be misconstrued to mean otherwise.

There may be risks associated with participating in activities mentioned in this book, for people in poor health or with pre-existing physical or mental health conditions. Because these risks exist, you should not participate in such diet plans if you are in poor health or have a pre-existing mental or physical condition. If you choose to follow any advice within this book, you do so of your own free will and accord, knowingly and voluntarily assuming all risks associated with such activities.

Facts and information are believed to be accurate at the time they were published in this book. All information provided is to be used for informational purposes only. Products and services described are only offered in jurisdictions where they may be legally offered. Information provided is not all-inclusive, and is limited to information that is made available. Such information should not be relied upon as all-inclusive or accurate.

You agree to hold South Peak Press, its owners, agents, and employees harmless from any and all liability for all claims for damages due to injuries, including attorney fees and costs, incurred by you or caused to third parties by you, arising out of the fitness and diet plans discussed in this book.

What You Need To Know About Getting In Shape

South Peak Press

CONTENTS

What You Need To Know About Getting In Shape

ACKNOWLEDGMENTS

Brian Copeland's Core Fitness, Aurora, CO
Coughlin Fitness & Results LLC, Washington, DC
Next Step Fitness, Champaign, IL
Impulsetraining.com, Canton, OH
Precision Health & Wellness, Carmel, IN
Home Bodies, Haverhill, MA
Never Give Up Fitness, Troy, MI
Rock Solid Personal Training Studio LLC,
Battle Creek, MI
IQ Fitness and Wellness, Atlanta, GA
Bootcamp-ct.com, Trumbull, CT
Beyond Expectations Coaching, VT
Your Fitness Your Life LLC, Boise, ID
Training Partners Inc., Asheville, NC
Golden Trainer Performance Studio Inc., Cedar Rapids, IA

INTRODUCTION

If you've ever spent any amount of time strolling through the "Fitness & Nutrition" books section at your local book store, you've probably noticed something: *there are so many books on the subject of losing weight and getting in shape!* While this large amount of information on the subject may seem like a good thing, it could also be the <u>one thing that keeps you from taking action</u> towards your personal fitness and nutrition goals.

Let me explain.

As you're probably aware, the fitness and nutrition industry is a multi-billion dollar industry. There are thousands upon thousands of "experts" who rely on you to buy the next fitness book, exercise gadget, or DVD that hits the store shelves or the late night TV airwaves. Unfortunately, in this profit-driven world known as the fitness and nutrition industry, one priority gets lost: getting real results for the end-user. You see, if one of these multi-million dollar companies actually produced a gadget or DVD that enabled everyone to be in the best shape of their lives forever, you wouldn't need to buy their products anymore - and that's exactly what they don't want to happen! Publishers and infomercial producers are profit-driven concerns after all. There has to be a "new and improved" version, a sequel, an "add-on," upgrade, or special offer *so they can take more money from you.* Remember this is BIG business. Huge amounts of money are made by providing you supposed solutions to your fitness and nutrition needs. Throw into this the facts that (1) health is an evolving science with knowledge in the field *doubling* every 2-3 years and (2) that each of us is unique with different needs and lifestyles and no wonder everyone is so confused about fitness and nutrition.

Ok, I know I'm being a bit cynical, but after working in the fitness and nutrition business for 20 years, I know what I'm talking about. But what does this mean for you? Should you just throw in the towel and give up on any and all information out there? Of course not. You do, however, need to be more selective about where you get your information.

That's where this book comes in.

The goal of this book was to interview **real** personal trainers who train clients **each and every day** of their professional lives. Inside this book you're not going to find interviews with celebrity fitness trainers. As you probably realize, most celebrity fitness trainers do very little day-to-day fitness training because it conflicts with their schedules of book signings, producing DVDs, and filming television commercials. It's sad to say, but many great personal trainers stop being great personal trainers the moment they get "discovered" by the marketing machine that is the fitness and nutrition industry.

Consider this book to be the opposite of those glitzy, celebrity-endorsed books. When we produced this book, we set out to find real world experts and that's exactly what we got. In fact, our biggest challenge was getting these personal trainers to break away from their busy schedules of training their clients, so that they could actually share their advice in this book! The trainers who have contributed to this book "walk the walk", and the content they've provided in the following chapters reflects their true practical knowledge and expertise. So turn off the TV, grab a pen a paper, and get ready to learn what you need to know to get in shape. Without further ado, we present to you the real world personal trainer interviews!

1 Brian Copeland

Do minors typically need to get the permission of an adult or guardian if they want to work with a personal trainer? If so, how does this work?

Any fitness, sports, or health professional will require some form of a "hold harmless" waiver from their clients. In the event of a minor, a guardian's signature would be required. Also, there is always some assumed risk when entering into sports or exercise so it would only be responsible to have the full support and understanding of the parents or guardian for the minor.

Why do some people lift heavy weights while other people lift lighter weights?

The reasons that some people lift heavier weights while others lift lighter weights are numerous. Some folks, such as competitive power lifters will lift heavy weights because that is the nature of their sport. Other individuals might lift light or heavy weights simply due to preference while still others will lift light or heavy based on what I like to call fitness mythology. Most people have been told that lifting heavy will make you big while lifting light will make you toned, that of course is a fallacy. It is generally understood in the world of exercise science that when someone lifts very heavy weights, say in the range of 1 - 3 repetitions, they are primarily going to create changes in their nervous system rather than build larger muscles, while this is not always the case it tends to hold true for most. Repetitions in the higher range, typically from 10 – 20, tend to promote changes in muscle size by creating more mitochondria and blood processing tissue. This is where people tend to "feel-the-burn" when they exercise. Repetitions in the in-between ranges 5 - 8 tend to offer a nice combination of neurological strength and muscle tone/size. By the way, when people desire to be more toned without getting big they often don't understand what "tone" really is. A toned body is one where the

3

visible curves of the muscle are showing. This can be achieved by either building more muscle, losing body fat so the muscle shows easier, or both. And doing both is the quickest route. For optimal health, general fitness enthusiasts should explore a variety of repetition ranges from heavy weight/low reps, to moderate reps and weight, all the way to lower weight and higher reps.

Do personal trainers normally work with clients who are only free on weekends or during off-hours? What's typical in terms of when personal trainers are available?

Typical personal trainers work with typical folks and typical folks work typical hours! Thus most personal trainers will find the bulk of their business during non-business hours, late afternoons, and early mornings. Many folks are not motivated to go see a trainer on the weekend, but a small group of dedicated folks will. Never forget that there are business owners, retirees and people who work non-traditional hours and days that are more than willing to seek personal training during typical work hours. I have several regular clients during the weekday afternoons.

If someone has back problems, or other physical limitations, how can they lift weights safely without getting hurt?

The most important thing that people need to understand is that a human body really, truly is difficult to injure. For someone who is coordinated, injury or pain during exercise is not normal. Having said that, most people are very uncoordinated with their own bodies yet want to jump right into a full-blast fitness program. According to a recent study, 80% of all new people who start a fitness program quit within the first 2 months due to injury! This is due to a poorly educated personal trainer and/or a gung-ho fitness enthusiast whose body is not yet ready for strenuous exercise. If you have been a couch potato for the last 10 years, you won't be Lance Armstrong in a week! Slow and steady is the smarter and safer way to go. I have a progressive system for training my clients and thus injuries are virtually nonexistent. For someone who is currently in pain, I highly recommend they seek a trainer who is educated in working with people in pain. Unfortunately, this type of trainer is very rare. The best people I have found in this area are called Z-Health Certified Performance Coaches.

Likewise, I am not a huge fan of one-sized-fits-all fitness classes and boot camps. I feel they force everyone to do the same work load and exercises and not everyone is ready for a certain amount of work and not all exercises are appropriate for everyone. People with limitations will find they can have a very fulfilling fitness program by finding the exercises that allow them to work around their limitation, and if their limitation is fixable then working to correct that issue should be top priority.

What is the typical way to pay a personal trainer? Weekly? Monthly? At each session?

Typically, personal training is purchased either in packages with a set number of sessions or in a monthly format, although many trainers will accept single session payments. Usually, a single session will come at a premium while a package or monthly rate will be offered at a discount.

When is a spotter needed for exercises?

In my professional opinion, I don't think the average fitness enthusiast should be doing an exercise that requires a spotter. The number of exercises that actually require a spotter I can count on one finger: the bench press. Any other exercise that someone performs should not be performed with a weight or level of resistance that the client does not have complete control over. Spotting may be required for individuals with low coordination, and/or vestibular and visual issues, who are prone to balance problems, but aside from that, if you need a spotter, I would stop and ask if you really should be lifting what you are lifting. There are certain athletes who may require a spotter or safety equipment due to the nature of their sport, for instance a very heavy bench press for a competitive power lifter. I favor kettlebells and body weight exercises for my clients as they require a mastery of their own bodies to perform them. Mastery of one's body is a good thing.

How does someone tone up in certain "problem areas?"

The term "problem area" can mean many things. Some examples of "problem areas" are: a mother has looser skin in her belly, a fairly thin person has a protruding belly, a woman with a slim-looking upper body carries a lot of weight in the hips, men with a saggy chest and women with "flying squirrel wings," as one of my female clients put it, under their upper arms. Problem areas are almost always due to excessive body fat and lack of muscle tone.

Diet and exercise will always help with these areas but here are a few tips:
1) Excessive belly fat - this is typically due to a stress hormone called

cortisol that likes to store fat in the belly. The best way to reduce this problem area is to take control of your life and reduce and/or deal with your stress, in addition to a healthy diet and exercise program.

2) Saggy areas (chest, upper arms, belly fat) - people use the term "problem area," but what they are seeing is also genetics: this is where your body likes to store body fat. Modern research says we cannot spot reduce fat in specific areas by exercising those areas. Body fat is lost overall in predetermined genetic patterns. So put the focus on just losing body fat, focus on controlling calories and eating healthier food. In addition, do strength/resistance training exercises for these areas to increase the muscle tone. Muscle and skin are connected via a soft tissue called fascia. Tone the muscles and the skin will hold onto more tone via the fascia that lies beneath.

3) Slim upper body and heavier lower body - Everything from lymphatic flow to genetics can affect your body type, but as with point (2) above, you can't spot reduce, so just focus on losing more body fat via healthy nutrition, controlling calories, and exercising your body with full-body exercises (e.g, squats instead of knee extensions, pull-ups instead of curls). Full-body exercises burn more calories and tone more muscles than just training single-muscle exercises.

Is it true that too much cardio can be unhealthy?

Interestingly, the research says "yes," too much cardio can be unhealthy. In fact, the Journal of Applied Physiology published a study demonstrating that excessive cardio caused increased myocardial scar tissue and increased risk of heart disease. Various other studies have shown the same. The question is, "what is too much cardio?" Then again, what exactly IS cardio?

Cardio is often associated with mild movement such as walking to more moderate activities such as cycling, jogging, swimming, using a treadmill, stairmaster or elliptical machine. However, these activities only work what is known as the "aerobic" cardio system. When you do a sprint on your feet or with a bicycle, you will feel your heart and lungs fatigue far faster. This is called "anaerobic" cardio. Aerobic cardio uses oxygen as the primary fuel source while anaerobic cardio uses sugar (knows as muscle glycogen) as the primary fuel source. In the event of a heart attack it is not aerobic cardio health that you need but anaerobic cardio. Anaerobic cardio forces your heart to deal with larger volumes of blood and oxygen, which is precisely what happens during a heart attack. Aerobic cardio doesn't really achieve this. However, while brief sessions of aerobic-zone cardio is not bad for you, excessive aerobic cardio is. Long distance marathon running, cycling and similar cause your heart to become weaker and build excessive scar tissue. Also, the sheer volume of work involving the heart from this type of activity causes chronic inflammation. Inflammation leads to muscle wasting and weakness. A small, weak heart is not "what the doctor ordered." In any major marathon in the United States there will be at least a handful of runners who drop dead of heart attacks. I've never heard of any other sport where that happens.

I'm not trying to scare you away from cardio, just realize that jogging for long distances is not really a healthy choice. Short distances is fine. By the way, any time you do any type of exercise where your blood pressure rises, respiration increases and heart rate increases, you are doing cardio. Toss a medicine ball at a wall 20 times, play a game of tennis, do 8 heavy barbell or kettle bell squats and you are doing heart-healthy cardio.

What are the benefits of hiring a personal trainer over just buying some DVDs that feature personal trainers?

There tend to be two camps of people: self-motivated and unmotivated. Self-motivated people are likely to buy a fitness DVD and stick to it. However, everyone else will buy a fitness DVD, maybe watch it a few times (or never) and that is the end of the story. Both types of individual would benefit from seeking out a fitness professional. The self-motivated person will benefit from finding an expert on the material on the DVD to ensure they are using proper form, truly understand the content, and are getting the most out of the product. People without motivation need another person to give them motivation. They need routine and to slowly build the habit of exercise. Believe it or not, motivation is actually a skill and you can get better at it by practicing it. People need to build the habit of exercise, see the benefits of what they are doing and then tie that into a deep emotional reason to exercise: et voila, motivation is being built.

Is it a good idea to walk or run with weights? Will this produce results quicker?

I do not endorse walking or running with weights for much distance. Everything must have a purpose and if there is not a specific purpose then don't do it. Walking is part of a reflexive gait pattern called inter limb neurocoupling reflex and is tied to something called central pattern generators. While all of this neurophysiology may sound like Greek, it is actually important to health and well-being. There are athletes such as strong man competitors who do what is called farmer's carries where they will pick up heavy objects and walk with them for 50 yards or so, I'm ok with that. But putting light dumbbells in your hands and walking for miles really doesn't burn any significant amount of calories anyway so why risk messing up your natural gait pattern? As far as running with weights, I'm not sure I can think of a reason to do that. To increase the vertical load does not make sense from an athletic perspective or calorie burning perspective. If someone wants to run fast a better idea is to study the Jamaican sprint team's mechanics, the top several fastest sprinters in the world come from the tiny little island of Jamaica. Why are they so fast? They have an amazing coach that teaches amazing sprint mechanics. Running with weights will actually force you to change your sprint mechanics to compensate for the weight and thus you will be slower when you take the weights away. Bad idea! If Usain Bolt, the fastest man in the world, does it, then go ahead, but he doesn't so neither should you.

How soon after someone starts a diet and exercise program should they start to see results? When will they know if their diet and exercise program is working?

Individuals vary greatly, but as a general rule the average person should notice results in their appearance in 12 weeks. Depending on their program and how closely they follow it they should notice other results much faster. This is why I recommend people take several types of measurements so they can see results, or a lack thereof, much sooner. The sooner someone gets feedback, the sooner they can change course or develop more motivation and belief in their hard work. Looking in the mirror is deceptive because 0.167 lbs of body fat per day doesn't really show well. But a body fat % scale, a tape measure, belt loops, etc. all give reliable and objective feedback. Relying on only "thinking" or "believing" that your diet and exercise program is or is not working is akin to never looking at your car's speedometer and just guessing how fast you are going as you drive past that state trooper. Bad idea! So don't "think" or "believe" that a program is working or not: track it using several objective measuring tools.

What are some of the most common misconceptions people have about hiring a personal trainer?

Well, I hate to say this, but a huge mistake is assuming that your personal trainer knows what they are doing. I heard someone once say that you should never pick a lawyer out of a phone book and I believe that same thing applies to any profession. I would interview a prospective personal trainer. Make sure that you have rapport with them. Do they know how to listen to your concerns and address them or do they just tell you what to do and seem oblivious to your needs? Do they have success stories? Do they look the part, walk-the-walk as it were? Unfortunately, many personal trainers have a weekend degree and a lack of true passion for what they do. Find someone passionate about fitness AND helping others. When someone is passionate they are more likely to continue their education. I always tell people to ask a prospective doctor what is the last book they read about their field. I want to know if a Doctor is stuck in medical school from 1960 or if they read newer research. Well, the same goes for a personal trainer.

What are some of the most common myths about nutrition?

Common myths about nutrition are numerous. There are probably more myths about nutrition than almost any other thing I have ever studied. Let's start with some controversial ones to make things fun. First one: dietary cholesterol and saturated fat are unhealthy for you. In fact, the opposite may well be true. Last year the National Association of Bariatric Doctors met to discuss a number of issues including the impact of dietary cholesterol and saturated fat on heart health. After all of the evidence was presented an interesting thing happened, there was no evidence at all! In fact, there has never been a single legitimate study that has linked a diet high in cholesterol and saturated fat to heart problems. In fact, the studies that have been done have shown that nations and cultures that eat a high fat, high cholesterol diet have the best longevity and heart health.

Next myth: a diet high in grains, breads, pasta, cereals, etc. are good for your health. Wrong! Whether you fall on the evolution or creation side of the coin, it is evident that human kind has been eating and is ideally suited to eat a diet high in animal meat, vegetables, fruits, nuts and seeds and virtually zero grains. That means deciding whether to get wheat bread or whole wheat bread is irrelevant, don't get either one. Starchy carbohydrates are cheap, low-quality, hard for humans to digest and spike our levels of the hormone insulin, which if spiked chronically leads to type 2 diabetes, obesity and a number of other health related illnesses including food allergies.

Another myth: taking your daily vitamin pills is a good idea. Wrong! Now for the record, I do believe in taking high quality vitamins, minerals, omega 3 fatty acids, etc. But the problem is that people buy cheaper grocery store brand supplements and those supplements are almost always made in China which has horrible quality control. Most of the time what is on the label is not what is in the pill. When purchasing vitamin supplements look for ones made from organic vegetables and fruits and also look for a quality control certification such as "GMP" or "made in an FDA certified facility."

What are some of the biggest mistakes that people make when they start an exercise program?

I see 3 big mistakes. The first is that people don't set clearly defined goals. I hear people say things like, "I want to get in shape." I usually tell them that they are already in "a shape" and ask them what sort of shape would they like to have. Without a clear picture of what they want to look like, perform like or feel like, how will they know if they are getting closer or not? I recommend finding a picture of someone from a fitness magazine or other place that looks like the body you want to have.

The second biggest mistake is they don't chose a form of exercise that will help them reach their goals. I have people tell me they want to put on muscle, lose body fat, perform better in their sport and look like a fitness model, all great goals. But then they tell me they have been doing daily jogging and are not happy with the results. Well, of course not! Take a look at the average jogger's body, take a look at a high-level marathon runner's body. That is not the same type of body this person just described they wanted. If you want to put on muscle and lose fat find the people with the body you want and find out what they did to get there. There are often multiple routes but you need to pick one of them that develops the body you want.

The third mistake is that people tend to jump in too fast and don't take the time to build fitness gradually. I am fond of telling people, "you have to get fit enough to get fit." What that means is that you need to get your joints mobile and strong enough to take the stress of more intense exercise. You need to get your mind and spirit conditioned enough to enjoy more intense exercise. When people push it too hard and too fast exercise feels unpleasant and they end up quitting. I'd rather someone not be allowed to exercise as hard as they want to, that way they are chomping at the bit for their next session. I usually tell people they have to earn the right to do more exercise. You would be amazed at how earning the privilege to exercise makes people do their homework, i.e., not miss exercise sessions or stay on track with their nutrition.

How does someone know how hard to push themselves when they're working out?

I love to tell people that "fitness is not punishment, it is something you do to help you reach your goals." Far too many people have been brainwashed into thinking "no-pain = no-gain." Well, that is absurd. Pain is a traumatic reaction to a negative event. So literally people will push through pain and discomfort and abuse themselves because they think it will get them better results. It doesn't.

First, if you dislike exercise you are less likely to stick with it. So, you MUST stop an exercise session while you still enjoy it.
Second, pushing too hard releases a stress hormone called cortisol. Cortisol stores body fat and blocks protein uptake into the muscle by as much as 70%. That means that if you exercise too hard you can burn muscle away and store body fat, the exact opposite of what you are trying to do! Third, my colleagues and I have a saying, "amazing athletes make really hard things look easy while average gym rats make really easy things look hard." I am amazed by the grace and calm faces of world-class Olympians who perform feats of athleticism that inspire. Then you go to any gym, USA and see someone doing the easiest exercise, such as a dumbbell curl, and their faces look like they are passing a kidney stone! If you look at world-class athletes they have the types of bodies people really want, so why not do what they do? My advice: stay calm, relaxed, exercise as long as you enjoy it. When you get burned out, tired, etc., it is time to quit your session. Give yourself permission to be able to end an exercise session whenever you want to and the next time you go to exercise you will be chomping at the bit instead of dreading it.

Brian can be reached at brian@bccorefitness.com
or Brian Copeland's Core Fitness, Aurora, CO

2 MARILYN MCALLISTER

Can people use an exercise ball if they are overweight or obese?

Exercise balls are excellent tools in the right application. However, they are air filled balls with a weight limit. If a person is overweight or obese, the ball will be compressed significantly when the person sits on the ball. The ball will not provide the support necessary to perform exercises correctly. An obese person could also become unstable and fall off the ball.

Exercise balls provide an unstable surface for performing many exercises. Research has shown that instability results in greater recruitment of core muscles (e.g. abdominals, low back, erector spine, hip stabilizers). This can be helpful as an exercise variation for the experienced exercise participant. However, the primary exercise focus for an overweight or obese person is to burn calories, preferably doing full body movement. Save the exercise balls until weight is reduced and exercise experience shows the person is ready for a new challenge.

Is it bad to eat right before going to bed? Why or why not?

Eating right before going to bed can contribute to acid reflux. Unmanaged acid reflux can lead to esophageal damage and potentially cancer. For this reason alone, eating a large meal or foods that cause acid reflux immediately before bedtime is inadvisable.

Eating a large meal right before going to bed can also disrupt sleep. Disrupted sleep patterns can lead to fatigue, weight gain, and other health concerns.

Usually when this question is asked, the concern is about body weight management. If the total calories consumed during the day are the same as the energy expended, the timing of the calorie intake does not appear to be important. Unfortunately, it's common for people to continue snacking into the evening even if their calorie needs have been met by the end of dinner. Late night snacking causes weight gain, not because of the time of day, but because the total calories for the day are too high.

What are some tips that people should keep in mind for practicing good form during their workouts?

Learning to maintain a neutral spine position is one of the most important exercise technique skills. A neutral spine position is the normal, upright position of the spine. When looking at a person from the side there should be slight curves: inward at the cervical spine, outward at the thoracic spine and back inward at the lumbar spine. Practice holding the spine neutral while performing exercise such as squats, lunges, lat pull-down, planks, crunches, and even walking.

Can someone still lose weight if they split their workouts throughout the day?

Research shows that the health and weight management benefits of exercise are a result of the physical activity accumulated throughout the day. Exercise can be done in short bouts throughout the day with great success. Every little bit is helpful including taking the stairs, parking farther away from the door to increase walking time, and walking or biking to do errands.

A person just getting started with an exercise program can be more successful if the work is split into manageable sessions through the day. Busy people may also have better success fitting in short workouts at home or at work rather than insisting on hour long sessions at a gym. This can be a wonderful strategy for many people who are working on weight loss.

How should the diet of someone who's looking to build muscle differ from the diet of someone who wants to lose weight?

To gain muscle you must eat enough calories to support the muscle building process. Daily calorie intake must be sufficient for all daily activities and the additional strength training required to build muscle. It's typical to add 200-500 calories per day to the diet as the strength training workouts increase to reach the muscle building goal. Protein intake may increase slightly, though this is often over stated. A protein intake of 1.4-2.0 grams of protein per kilogram of body weight is quite sufficient to support muscle growth.

To lose weight you must burn more calories than you eat. For weight loss we recommend creating a calorie deficit of about 500 calories per day. This deficit should be created by a combination of increasing exercise and decreasing total calories. Emphasizing low calorie vegetables and high fiber foods helps keep you feeling full with fewer calories.

What is the customary procedure, with regard to payment, if someone has to cancel an appointment with their personal trainer?

Most personal trainers have a cancellation policy. At our studio, we request 24 hour notice for cancellations or rescheduling. If an appointment is cancelled inside that 24 hour window the client pays for the cancelled or missed session.

How long after eating should people wait to work out?

You shouldn't be either full or hungry when you exercise. How much time you wait after eating depends on what and how much you have eaten. It maybe 3-4 hours after a big meal before you feel comfortable to exercise. However, a light snack such as a piece of fruit can be perfect just 30 minutes before exercise. It also depends on what type of exercise you'll be doing. Many people can go for a brisk walk soon after eating; however, they may need to wait much longer if they are going to be running.

What should someone bring with them to a personal training session?

All you need at a personal training session is a good attitude, a little of your own motivation and comfortable clothing. The personal trainer should have water available as well as any equipment you'll need.

How should people with asthma approach their workouts?

People with asthma should always check with their physician prior to starting an exercise program. Your physician should provide guidelines for exertion and instructions about what to do if you have an asthma episode while exercising. You need to share this information with your personal trainer so that he or she can also be prepared.

What are some examples of foods that people think are good for them, but they're really not, and why are these foods actually not healthy?

Packaged foods such as nutrition bars, protein shakes and other meal replacements are the most misunderstood food items. They are processed foods labeled to make us believe that they are better than real, simple, fresh foods. Processing almost always takes away important nutrients that existed in the natural food.

Is it true that it becomes harder to lose weight as people get older? If so, why?

Weight management becomes harder with age for many people. While we like to blame age by itself, usually weight gain is a result of moving less and eating too much. If you can continue a vigorous exercise program, it is unlikely that weight management will be a problem. However, many people do experience effects of aging, such as arthritis, that make it difficult to maintain a vigorous exercise program. If this is the case, food intake must decrease to match the reduced activity.

What types of scheduling commitments are customary when hiring a personal trainer? In other words, do people normally take things one week at a time or are they typically asked to schedule several weeks at a time with their trainer?

There are a variety of scheduling methods used by personal trainers. Our studio prefers to schedule for a month in advance. However, we allow flexibility to change and experiment with schedules so we can find the schedule that works best for each client. Since we are educators and coaches, we have clients who meet with us up to five times per week and others who come in just once a month.

Payment is always made in advance for the sessions scheduled in the coming month at our studio.

If someone has a favorite food that they could never give up forever, what do you suggest?

We don't classify any food as totally off limits. If a client has a favorite food that is particularly unhealthy we help them gradually reduce the frequency and quantity of that food. We help them see how a small serving of that food can fit in the overall calories they need. Completely avoiding a favorite food will only make you crave it more.

Is it true that people can exercise their abs every day? Will this speed up their results?

Core muscles can be worked more often than three times a week. However, working them every day never gives them time to recover. Three to five times a week might be reasonable. Whether or not this schedule will speed up results depends not just on frequency but also on the intensity and quality of the core work being done.

Is it better for someone to workout at home or at a gym with their personal trainer? What are the pros and cons to each?

This is a completely personal choice. Ask yourself:

Where am I most likely to make the appointments and get the work done?

Where am I most comfortable?

Where do I feel that I get the best workout?

What situation will help make me successful?

Marilyn McAllister, Owner of Your Fitness Your Life, Boise, ID, can be reached at marilyn@yourfitnessyourlife.com or 208 841 5433

3 JIM COUGHLIN

Is it true that men should lift heavier weights and women lighter weights?

People who lift heavy weights are typically trying to put on muscle mass and build strength whereas people who lift lighter weights are trying to maintain the muscle they have and basically strengthen muscle imbalances, but this question tends to be misinterpreted when it comes to women. Most women think that if they lift very heavy, they're going to get big and muscular like men. But this is simply not the case. Women do not have as much testosterone as men and therefore will only develop a lean muscular body. They will not develop the size that their male counterparts will. Having said that, if a woman has a high percentage of body fat and does a strength training/weight lifting program with heavy weights and low reps, while neglecting cardiovascular exercise and proper nutrition, she may develop the appearance of being bulky. This is because the muscle underneath the fat is causing the area to expand because the fat is not being burned off properly. This is a very complex question to answer and can be more thoroughly explained as a woman starts to go through her exercise program with a trainer.

How can you tell if you're getting a sufficient workout?

With strength training you usually will feel a strong burn due to lactic acid building up in your muscles as you reach your last rep. This tells you that you are pushing your muscles to their max. With cardio, there are two ways to know you are pushing yourself hard. One is the Karvonean formula, which is 220 - age = your maximum heart rate. From this number you can monitor your intensity by doing your cardio at a 50-85% intensity range. Obviously, the higher the number, the harder you are working. The other is the talk test. If you can talk easily you are not working hard enough. If you find it difficult to talk you are working too hard.

Can children/teenagers benefit from working with a personal trainer?

Yes, absolutely. Implementing an exercise and nutrition program into your life is more complex than most people realize. Before starting, it's imperative that a minor be put through a very thorough examination of their health history to ensure they are safe to exercise. Also, in addition to the exercise sessions that a trainer will put the minor through, it's very important for the minor's guardian to make sure the minor follows through with necessary nutritional guidelines set forth by the trainer and/or nutritionist/dietician. A minor's body is going through huge changes and if they only do the exercise sessions while neglecting proper nutrition, they will easily start to develop deficiencies, and this could result in more harm than good.

Will a trainer help me with each exercise and every rep?

It really depends. If you're asking about the personal training, a trainer spots a client with practically every exercise to ensure he/she is safe and is using proper form. But if someone were to be exercising alone, you really don't need a spotter, contrary to what many experts say. My belief is if you know how to perform an exercise and you know how many reps and how much weight you should be doing, you should know what your limits are. So that means if you feel that doing 3 more repetitions of a particular exercise will put you in an unsafe situation, you simply don't do them. If you are using momentum and bad form with an exercise then that means the weight is too heavy and you should reduce it. To build muscle, your muscles must experience controlled tension, so a spotter is basically unnecessary when you have complete control of your exercise movements.

I'm okay everywhere else, but I'd really like to get rid of my belly fat. Can a personal trainer help?

Ahh...I knew this question was coming. Spot reducing is simply not possible. The best way I can describe this is by telling you how your body changes as you exercise and eat healthy. When you strength train your body is breaking down and building lean muscle. When you perform cardiovascular exercise your body is burning off excess fat. When you eat consistently healthy your body is replenishing itself with the proper nutrients it needs to help repair your muscle and also burn of excess fat. All 3 of these factors must be incorporated in order for your body to change. But your body changes as a whole, not just in one particular problem area, or as I like to tell clients, "Your body burns fat globally, not locally." If someone is unhappy with a particular problem area, they must be patient and understand that eventually, if they do everything correctly with their exercise and nutritional regimen, the fat will decrease in those areas.

I've heard that too much cardio can lead to muscle loss. Is that true?

Sometimes too much cardio can cause people to lose muscle which eventually can lead to being unhealthy, but it's only when the cardio is something extreme and the exerciser is not eating properly such as running marathons. The most cardio I recommend to clients and what I also do myself, is twice a day for no more than an hour at a time. I tell them also to space it out, performing one session in the morning and one in the evening. That way your body gets proper nourishment in between sessions. If you lift weights on a given day, I recommend doing cardio only once while also spacing both exercise sessions out.

Should a person avoid weights if they have a weakness due to injury, some other limitation, or pain?

The job of the trainer is to strengthen a client's weaknesses while simultaneously working around their physical limitations. The best way for someone to lift weights safely without getting hurt is to use proper form with each exercise while also using the correct amount of weight. If a particular exercise begins to cause some type of pain, then you should immediately stop and try something different.

There are a lot of DVDs that feature personal trainers teaching workouts. Can't I just use them instead of a live personal trainer?

Well, the motivation and accountability are the biggest benefit that comes along with hiring a personal trainer. DVDs are helpful; however, the individual still has to force himself/herself to do the exercises, whereas with a live training you don't have a choice! Monitoring exercise design, form, reps, weight, nutrition, etc. are also huge benefits to hiring a real personal trainer because they can create a program tailored exactly to your fitness level. DVDs tend to be a more generic, one-size-fits-all for exercise design. So while they are helpful, they aren't as valuable as hiring a real trainer.

I'm tired of waiting so long to get results. How can I reach my goals faster?

My clients usually see results after a couple weeks, but it also greatly depends on the client. If an individual is doing everything I tell them to do with their cardio and nutrition and also doing their best with me when I meet with them, then they will reap the benefits and get results the quickest. However, the individuals who are slacking in a particular area and not working as hard as they can with me, are going to experience results at a slower rate. Everything you do matters and you don't want to leave something to chance. Some individuals may have a higher metabolism then others, but I still think that everyone has the ability to be in phenomenal shape and maximize their full potential.

My cousin knows a lot about fitness. Why shouldn't I save money and listen to her instead of hiring a personal trainer?

Probably the biggest misconception people have is that a personal trainer isn't worth the investment. The reason people think this is because many people have never taken exercise and eating healthy seriously, so they don't see the value in hiring a personal trainer. Like anything in life, you usually experience success if you enlist in expert advice or receive expert help. Would you trust yourself working on your own car if something was wrong with it or would you get the help of a mechanic? Would you represent yourself if you had a conflict with the law or would you hire an attorney? Exercise and eating healthy is no different. It's a very complex subject and there is no reason you shouldn't seek out an expert to achieve the best results.

Unfortunately, many trainers aren't as knowledgeable and as passionate as others and tend to do it part-time. So in some cases a person who hires a part-time trainer is receiving a false representation of what they actually should be getting if they were to instead hire one who trains full-time and takes things more seriously.

When it comes to payments, how do personal trainers charge for their services?

Usually clients pay for a package deal up front (2 months of training 3x-5x a week) to prove they are committed. However, my company also allows you to make weekly or monthly payments if you can't afford to pay for everything at once.

What might beginners do wrong when they start a training program.

They start off too strenuously and burn themselves out and/or possibly injure themselves. They also have unrealistic expectations of what type of results they can expect to achieve.

Will a personal trainer work with my schedule, say early mornings or even weekends, or do I have to conform to the gym schedule?

A full time personal trainer is available at any time to train when a client wants to. But typically, since most working professionals work 9-5 jobs, trainers usually train them early in the morning (5am-8am) or late at night (5pm-8pm), or as you said, on the weekends.

----

*Jim Coughlin is personal trainer and fitness author for Coughlin Fitness & Results. He trains clients in their homes, offices or eligible gyms in the Washington DC metro area. You can visit his website at www.fitnessandresults.com or you can contact his company at **1-866-255-8221** to set up a free consultation.*

4 STEVE GRATKINS

Is it a bad idea to eat right after working out? Why or why not?

It's a great idea to have a nutritional source after a workout. I recommend having a recovery drink made up of carbohydrates, protein, and fat. The best drink for your money is a glass of 1% chocolate milk 15 to 30 minutes after your workout. After one to two hour of taking your recovery drink (chocolate milk) you should have a wholesome meal. The wholesome meal should be made with lean proteins, complex carbohydrates, and unsaturated and saturated fats. Good examples would be chicken with Mediterranean rice and vegetables, a turkey sandwich on whole wheat bread served with spinach, sprouts, tomatoes, onions, and low fat condiments.

What should someone do if they get muscle cramps during a workout? Should they work through it or do something else?

It depends on what type of exercise the person is doing. If a person is running and they get "stitches," a cramp in the ribcage area, they should slow down, drink water, and ensure they are breathing at a controlled pace with their back straight. If a person is weight lifting or running and their calf muscle starts to cramp, they should stop the activity, massage the area, stretch, and drink water. People need to remember to drink water throughout the day, during their workout, and after their workout. This will help maximize their potential and prevent cramping.

How can someone tell if their personal trainer's certification is legitimate?

Good question. There are too many certifications. The biggest names are National Strength and Conditioning Association (NSCA), American College of Sports Medicine (ACSM), National Academy of Sports Medicine (NASM), and American Council on Exercise (ACE). It's also a good idea to find out what kind of educational background the trainer has. Many of the best trainers have advanced college education in kinesiology. Some of the degrees in this field may include exercise science, exercise physiology, biomechanics, and athletic training.

Is there any true benefit to warming up, cooling down, or stretching before or after exercising? If there is, why are these things important?

Yes, these are important activities to do. We need to define the two different types of stretching which the average person should perform. These types are Static and Dynamic Stretching. Static stretching can be described as a prolonged hold of a muscle in a stationary position. An example would be a quad stretch where you stand on one foot and lift your opposite foot's ankle to your butt and hold the stretch for 15 seconds. Dynamic stretching is best described as large, slow and controlled movement throughout the full range of motion of a joint. A good example would be arm circles.

Dynamic stretching should be performed at the beginning of a workout. It promotes the flow of blood to muscles and synovial fluid in the joints. Then walking on a treadmill or riding a bike at a slow pace for five to ten minutes will also help you prep the body for exercise. After your workout static stretching should be done. This type of exercise will help promote muscle regeneration and prevent muscle soreness. All muscle groups which were used during the workout should be stretched at the end of the workout.

Why is it important for people to work on improving their balance and how can they do this?

Some of the biggest physical problems a person may have stem from muscle imbalances. Many people in today's society spend long hours sitting in a desk. This position over a prolonged period of time can force the chest and hip flexor muscles to become much stronger than their opposite muscle actions. Having a muscle imbalance in these areas can force the upper back to bend forward, arms to twist thumbs in toward the body, and can result in low back pain. By working with a trainer or having a proper training program you can train your body to have perfect muscle balance and this will help eliminate body pains.

What are some of the most common myths about losing weight?

The biggest one I hear is that carb's are bad! This is completely false. Carbohydrate is your body's preferred fuel source at high intensity and is the only source of fuel for your brain. A health body needs an adequate balance of Carbs, Proteins, and Fats. Carbs should make up about 55 to 60 % of your diet and should be from complex carbohydrates sources such as brown rice, whole wheat breads and whole grain pastas. Most fruits and vegetables are also good. Try to limit your intake of foods which are highly processed such as white bread and white rice. Protein intake should be about 15% of your total calories. Protein should come from foods with as little fat in them as possible. Good examples of protein are lean beef, chicken, or fish. None of your protein sources should be fried. Fats should comprise about 15 to 30% of your diet. You should eat both saturated and unsaturated fats. When choosing fats, try olive oil for cooking, avocados, and lean red meats. Remember to avoid trans-fatty acids and partially hydrogenated oils.

Another common myth is that you can target fat loss. You can't! Subcutaneous body fat is nothing more than stored energy. When you combine aerobic and strength training while eating a proper diet, you will lose fat and gain lean muscle all over your body.

What is the correct way to breathe when working out?

When strength training, you need to breathe when your body is working. An example would be if you're doing a bench press. During the push phase you need to exhale and inhale when lowering the weights. Another example is lat pull downs. When pulling you need to exhale and inhale when raising your arms. The biggest thing to remember is to keep breathing and not hold your breath! Holding your breath can cause your blood pressure to skyrocket.

When doing aerobic exercise the most important thing is to get air in your lungs. You don't need to breathe in through your nose and out through your mouth. When your body is working hard in needs oxygen and it will not discriminate about where it comes from! Breathing at a controlled and comfortable pace with your back straight will help you perform aerobic exercise.

If a particular exercise hurts, is that normal?

If you are feeling pain you need to stop doing that exercise. You may feel a slight discomfort when exercising that passes after you're done. That is normal. However, if you feel sharp pain or a very uncomfortable feeling you need to stop that exercise. You may want to talk to the staff at the gym or a doctor to see what you should do or stop doing.

What are the must-have items that someone should bring with them to a personal training session?

Gym clothing, a water bottle, and a positive attitude.

What is "core strength"?

The core is comprised of all the muscles around your abdomen and back. You can think of the core muscles as a weight belt and how it's used to hold everything together. Core strengthening exercised can be anything from back hyperextensions to sit ups and plank exercises. You can add these exercises to your workout or you can do aerobic, or yoga classes to strengthen this group of muscles.

If someone spent the day doing something very strenuous like mountain biking or hiking, should they take a day off before working out or does the other activity not count as a real workout?

Yes, it is fine to take a day off from working out, or do a light workout instead. The thing about taking a day off is that you are making an excuse not to be physically active and this is bad. You need to be physically active on most, if not all, days of the week. Maybe just go for a long walk around the block, or if you're strength training do two sets instead of three. If you continue to be physically active every day, you're building a habit of exercise and instilling a lifestyle change which will pay off in the long run.

Is there an "ideal" time of day to work out?

I like to work out early in the morning because I get it done at the beginning of my day. The longer you put off working out throughout the day the easier it is to make an excuse not to exercise. If you are someone who can go to the gym every day after work then you don't need to do this, but making regular daily exercise a routine is a necessity. Also, try to write it down in your calendar to help hold you accountable.

Is it true that genetics or body physiology make it impossible for some people to get in shape?

It is true that genetics and past lifestyle choices can make it harder to get in shape. People need to also not set unrealistic goals. Most guys will never look like Brad Pit in Fight Club and most women will not look Jessica Alba in Sin City. If you're looking to lose weight, a healthy weight loss goal should be about one to two pounds every week. Any more can be unhealthy and is usually unsustainable. Also, keep in mind that you did not put weight on overnight, so don't expect to lose weight overnight - it takes time. A good goal for someone wanting to lose ten pound would be... "I will lose ten pounds in seven to eleven weeks." Write down your goal, make it visible to you every day, don't cheat yourself, and attack your goal.

How can people accurately determine how many calories they burn during a workout?

We are very lucky to live in an age of technology. Counting the calories you burn at the gym is important, but counting the calories you burn outside of the gym is more important. I highly recommend buying a body monitor from 'body media.' You wear their armband on your upper arm and it counts how many calories you burn throughout the day. By knowing how many calories you burn and the number of calories you consume you can set achievable and realistic goals.

What is the "fat burning zone" that trainers often refer to?

Many trainers talk about fat burning zones. This type of terminology is used far too often and it should stop. The goal should be to get someone to enjoy their workout program and get them to commit to a long-term lifestyle change.

While there are heart rate zones where the body will use fat as a fuel source more than carbohydrates, you don't need to keep your heart rate in these zones all the time. If you are in a fat burning zone your body will not burn as many calories after exercise compared to high intensity exercise which, during the exercise, will burn mainly carbohydrates as a fuel sources. If you wanted a good estimation of your heart rate zones take (220 - your age) x (.05 to .65) for fat burning zone or (220 - your age) x (.75 to 1.00) for carbohydrate burning zone.

What should someone look for in a good health club/gym?

Look for things that you would like to do. If you want personal training, look to see if personal trainers are at the club. If you want group classes look to see if the club has free classes with their membership or if you need to pay for them. Also, see if they have the type of classes you would like. An example would be, if you're a guy, you may not want to go to "Flirty Girl Fitness." A kick boxing class might suit you better. Maybe you want a spinning class. Joining a gym that does not offer this might not be for you. If you're a swimmer join a gym with a pool. Basically, look for what you want and you'll get what you want.

How can people tell if they're doing enough exercise or exercising intensely enough?

The American College of Sports Medicine (ACSM) recommends that you get one hour of aerobic exercise on most days of the week and that you engage in full body strength training on at least two days a week. If you can't do this because of your fitness level set a goal to work up to this. Try engaging in two ten-minute bouts of aerobic exercise four days a week and two days of full body strength training. If you are already at ACSM recommendations for exercise then try adding more aerobic or more strength training to your weekly regimen. After you are meeting the requirements you need to find an activity that you enjoy and that you can do continually. For me it's running marathons and commuting by bicycle during the warmer months.

How important is flexibility when it comes to getting in shape? Why is this important?

It is important to be flexible. You should be able to have full range of motion in all your joints. If your range of motion is limited in a joint, resistance training and stretching will help increase your flexibility. Talking to a personal trainer, physical therapist, or doctor will give you better insight about what exercises and stretches you should be performing.

How can personal trainers design programs for people with arthritis or others who are unable to perform certain common exercises?

Recent studies have shown that people suffering with arthritis can live with a better quality of life if they exercise. This appears to be due to increased mobility. While people with arthritis may not ever perform Olympic lifts, they can start out by training in a pool doing water aerobics, doing body weight exercises, using bands and light weights. Almost everyone can receive benefits from exercise such as increase endurance, strength, and flexibility.

How can people prevent joint injuries or sore joints when lifting weights?

The best way to prevent joint injuries is to not go beyond your normal range of motion, to exercise with a reasonable weight, and to keep the weights moving at a slow and controlled pace.

You can reach Steve at Steve@NextStepFitness.net

or 312-636-6861

5 TONYA ROCHO

Is it better to lift weights with free weights or with weight machines?

That would depend on the individual, their goals, physical abilities and their ability to execute proper exercise technique. Regardless of which one a person chooses to use, if the individual does not know how to engage the correct muscle intended to be worked and have proper form/technique, it can be a waste of time and very frustrating for the individual to reach their goal.

Why is one better than the other?

Free weights, in my opinion, are better.

The problem with machines is they are not designed for every body size and type. If a person is too small or too big for the machines, they will not be able to set up in proper posture to execute proper technique for the selected exercise. This will more than likely cause an injury or over-stress a muscle or joint, which can feel like an injury. If a person who is new to exercise joins a gym and is left on their own to figure out how to use the machines, they will more than likely have no idea how to set the machine for themselves and will just sit down and start using it, which can set a person up for injury. The instructions on the machines are not always the best explanation for someone who has no idea what they are doing. Machines also neglect the most important part of movement, the core. When a person sits in a machine they immediately rest their back on the back rest which relaxes all the important muscles that start movement. Research is showing that machines can actually make a user weaker and less functional, which leads to more injuries. Free weights can also have their drawbacks, but if taught proper form and technique a person can get more from their exercise in less time because they are recruiting more muscles and also placing more demand on their cardiovascular system which will also get them faster results.

Is it true that eating too many vegetables will make most people gain water weight?

That would depend on their source, fresh or canned. Canned vegetables are usually loaded with sodium and other preservatives that will cause water weight, but if you eat FRESH vegetables you will not gain water weight.

How can someone do resistance training if they don't own weights or belong to a gym?

Body weight work is better than weights and a gym. I believe if a person can master weight training with their own body weight, they will most certainly be stronger than the person who lifts weights. It is easy to push and pull weight but it is much harder to move yourself around and to hold yourself up.

Do people really lose muscle as they get older? If so, how much muscle do they lose on average and can anything be done to slow down this process?

Yes, people most certainly do lose muscle as they age. Depending on the person, 2%-3% can be lost on average per year. Proper nutrition and resistance training can slow down this process. Most people, not just the elderly, don't realize they are not getting enough food. They are bombarded with "eat less" and don't even realize that cutting calories too much can cause such a deficit that the body will rely on its own muscle (breaking it down) for energy. Medications can also cause muscle loss. It is best that a person consult with a professional to help them determine what is causing the muscle loss and then get them started in the right direction for an exercise and eating plan. There is way too much questionable information out there and most people do not fully understand what they are reading and how to apply it in their life to reach their goals.

How can someone figure out how many calories they should be eating each day?

Well, that can be tricky. A person can find a baseline by using any of the available calculators online, but it does not account for "who that person is and what they do". Most people also don't understand that when their body composition changes, their calorie needs will change as well. It is really important for a person to find a professional that understands this and can help them find their calorie needs for "who they are" and then to help monitor them to let them know when it is time to change their calories so they don't end up heading back to where they started.

Is it true that muscle will turn to fat if someone stops working out?

No. If you see someone that used to be muscular and now they appear to be fat, it's not because the muscle turned into fat, it's because the person stopped working out but didn't change his eating habits, so now that person added fat on top of the muscle. It could also be the person is no longer eating enough protein to support the muscle they once had, so now the body may be using the muscle for some energy. When that happens lean mass will go down and the fat mass will go up, but again, the muscle itself did not turn into fat.

What is "body fat percentage"? How does this differ from "body mass index"?

Body fat percentage is a measurement of how much fat a person has on their body. The percentage will encompass good fat and body fat and most forms of measurements will not break it down. There are forms of measurements that will, but you will need to see a professional that has the equipment to measure both good and bad fat. It is more accurate to measure body fat for health concerns than body mass index, because body mass index does not discern between lean mass and fat mass. To get an individual's BMI you divide height by weight, but where does it tell you how much is lean tissue? Is the lean tissue muscle, organs or bones? We just don't know. Example, if you have a 5'10" female that weighs 160 pounds with 20% body fat and you have another female that is 5'10" that weighs 160 pounds with 36% body fat, who would be healthier? If you figure their BMI (height divided by weight) they will come out the same. Clearly the first female will be leaner and healthier than the second one, who because of the higher body fat percentage, will be at risk for more diseases and chronic health issues down the road.

What can thin people do to build muscle?

Hire someone who can help them customize a plan just for them. The information world is full of ideas that may help a thin person build muscle, but without knowing more information about the individual, it is hard to tell readers how to accomplish their goals. We are all reading the information provided by so many different professionals, and it can get confusing. How does the average person decipher all the information to make it fit them? They can't. The information is like a suit – one size does NOT fit all. How does the reader know if they fit or not?...they don't. They just try, fail and give up.

Can couples or groups of people work out with a personal trainer at the same time?

Yes, and I find my couples and small groups have the most fun. They are having so much fun they don't even realize how hard they just worked out. Also, it is nice to have the additional motivation in the room. The energy is high and the workouts are effective.

If someone hasn't worked out in years, how should they get started in the safest way possible?

They should consider themselves a newbie even if they have past knowledge or experience. A lot can change and even though you don't feel your body has changed much, you might be very surprised how it has. There is nothing wrong with starting over, so put the ego aside, don't think you know everything, and get started on the right track to stay injury free.

Is it safe to workout first thing in the morning, on an empty stomach?

It's really an individual thing. I know what research and other professionals will say, but I know for myself, I cannot workout with anything in my stomach. I use a pre-workout drink but I do not drink a shake or eat any food because it slows me down and makes me feel very weak and heavy. This is where a trainer can help a person determine what is best for them. A trainer can help the person read what their body is saying and interpret it to keep training safe and to ensure the person is getting everything they need for their workouts.

Do personal trainers usually have insurance?

Yes. If they are working for a company, gym or just for themselves, they should have insurance. I do not recommend anyone train with a trainer who does not have insurance.

How can people, with very busy work schedules and family commitments, fit working out into their schedule?

Everyone has 30 minutes somewhere in their schedule. It is just a matter of realizing how important exercise is for them to fit in their schedule. When something is really important, there is always time for it, but you must first find the value for you in it.

How many grams of fat should people consume each day if they want to lose weight?

I would stay around 30g to 40g a day, BUT, everyone is different and their nutritional needs will be different. Here is one problem we have in the information world, everything is a blanket for everyone, but everyone does not fit under the blanket. This is why you should start off working with a professional. They can help you determine everything you need to be successful, from eating to exercising, based on YOUR needs and goals.

What are some of the most common myths about building muscle?

1. Lifting heavy weight will build bulky muscles, which is so untrue. Unless you are genetically gifted or you are taking illegal substances, it takes a long time to build muscle, let alone bulky muscles. Ladies really have nothing to worry about. Women need to lift heavy to get that sleek, tight and toned body that most want. 2. Building muscle takes hours of training. Actually, you will tear the muscle down training for hours, especially if you are not eating to accommodate the hours of training. 3. You have to be in pain the next day from your training session. Some tightness and soreness is normal, but if a person hurts with movement and stretch, then it is more than likely they over did it and did damage - not good because now scar tissue will form.

Tonya can be reached at

Rock Solid Personal Training Studio, LLC
1332 E Columbia Ave
Battle Creek, MI 49014
269-420-6582 (Office)
269-288-0406 (Fax)
www.rocksolidptstudio.com
mobile site:http://m.wix.com/tonyamarshall/rocksolidptstudio

6 PAUL RODGERS

Does it make a difference if someone just does all of their exercise over the weekend as compared to spreading it out over the week?

For some people the "weekend warrior" mentality is the only thing that works in their schedule, but this type of training can lead to repeated injuries, a low performance rate and less than optimal success with regard to fat burning.

How often should someone work out with a personal trainer?

Our ancestors were hunter gatherers who would not have survived without hard work, speed, strength and agility. Our modern day exercise programs should mimic this type of functional lifestyle. Most of our clients train with us 4-5 times a week and we give them financial incentives to make this fit into their budget. For those whose schedule does not allow this type of commitment we design a program that they can do by themselves.

Is coffee bad for someone who's trying to lose weight or get in shape?

One cup of coffee a day will probably not harm you and some research even suggests that there may be some benefits to small amounts of coffee. Ergogenic aids are any external influences that can be determined to enhance performance and although coffee can be listed in this category, it may be detrimental to weight loss. Caffeine is the most widely used drug in the world and because the profits from this industry are so great the industry can promote just about any health benefits they want to and they have the ability to finance a study to prove it. I believe that the biggest detriment to consumption of more than a cup of coffee a day is what it can do to a healthy diet. Coffee can reduce your appetite, but that's not always a good thing. Our bodies need nutrient dense foods. These foods not only help us maintain a healthy weight but they can also give us the energy that we need to get through our day and help fight disease.

Coffee and other stimulants can distract us from an appetite for healthy, nutrient dense foods.

How can a personal trainer help a client with regard to nutrition?

Let's face it, most personal trainers received their certification from a weekend seminar. Most of them have no business giving any nutritional advice and in most states it's illegal for them to prescribe a diet. There is a trainer on the "Biggest Loser" that recommends a Red Bull before every workout. "Nuff said"

Is it unhealthy to eat a vegetarian or vegan diet that has no meat or dairy?

I have been studying nutrition for over 40 years. At 16 I went on a vegan diet, and although not totally a vegan, I abstained from red meat for over 20 years. This was a mistake for me and I believe that it is a mistake for most people. 20% of the teeth on our mouth are canine teeth. I believe that we were meant to eat meat, however commercial meat is loaded with chemicals and is generally lacking in nutrients. Since I started eating meat again I have never had a piece of meat that is not organic and grass fed. If someone has a religious or moral need to be a vegetarian or a vegan I suggest they study the subject to make sure they are getting all the nutrients they need.

Once someone begins working out with a personal trainer, what goes on during the sessions?

Our training protocol is called Assessment Based Functional Integrated Training. After a careful assessment that looks for muscle and anatomical imbalances we design an individualized program that encompasses flexibility, strength and endurance. Every month our clients are assessed again and their individualized program is changed to match their needs.

How long should a personal training session last?

At our facility our sessions are 60 minutes. We believe that this amount of time is the most beneficial for weight loss and heart health.

How much will it cost to hire a personal trainer?

Our private sessions range between $75 and $100 an hour but at our facility we specialize in small group training (3-4 people in a group). This type of training is fun, safe, effective and affordable. These sessions are $30.

Is it better to work out for a long period of time at a low intensity or a short period of time at a high intensity?

Our Assessment Based Functional Interval Training protocol utilizes short bursts of low, moderate, and high intensity functional movements and continues for an hour in duration. During this time we typically will increase a person's heart rate to between 60% and 72% of their HRM (heart rate max) between 8-10 times in the hour. After each of these intervals we let their heart rate recover down to at least 45% of their HRM.

How do people get rid of loose skin after weight loss?

Healthy skin depends much more on our diet than it does on fancy lotions and creams. I once asked a beautiful 70 year old East Indian woman how she kept her skin so young and she described how she rubbed coconut oil over her body before showering and lightly padded herself partially dry afterward with a towel. I have used and recommended this technique ever since with amazing results.
Our skin is approximately 70% water, 25% protein and 2% lipids. Proper hydration and fat content are the two most important dietary factors that can aid to healthy and resilient skin. What are your main sources of hydration? If your answer is diet soda, coffee and juice your body and your skin are in desperate need of hydration. If you drink fresh spring water from glass containers and put water filters on your showers you are doing just about the best you can do for your skin as far as hydration.

Our bodies know what to do with real fat. Among other things it stores fat as an energy source and it uses it for cell rejuvenation, including the cells of our skin. The best dietary fats are found in foods that we would have been able to find 5,000 years ago. Included in this category are animal fats and fats from vegetables/ fruits/seeds such as avocados and coconuts.

How do people measure their heart rate?

At our facility we recommend that most people over 45 use a heart rate monitor. For those who do not use a heart rate monitor we recommend either a 6 second or a 10 second count. These are accurate and time efficient. The most common site is the bottom of the wrist at the radial artery. The 6 second count is multiplied by 10 and the 10 second count is multiplied by 6.

Why is it that no matter how much cardio some people do they still can't

lose weight?

Just doing cardio is not always the fastest road to weight loss. Increasing muscle mass and adding intervals will get you there much faster. So far in my practice I have found that as long as someone has the physical ability to burn more than 3,500 calories a week and they can change their diet to my recommendations they will be successful in finding their genetic weight. The press and media push forward an unrealistic view of a physical appearance that they consider beautiful and healthy. I think one potential problem that occurs is when people want to go below their genetic weight. I believe that some people have more of a toxic load than others and this can affect their liver, slow their metabolism, and slow the weight loss.

Do men lose weight faster than women?

Yes, men do lose weight faster than women. They have bigger engines which consume more gas. Men have larger amounts of calorie-burning muscle mass on their frames and metabolically speaking, muscle tissue burns more stored fat than any other tissue or organ. For many reasons, especially to do with child bearing and nourishment of children, women are predisposed to store more fat.

Is there an ideal time of day to work out?

The best answer for this question depends on a lot of factors, especially the specific goals of the client. Scientific research suggests that afternoon workouts are slightly safer and performance is slightly higher, but I have always attributed my high success rate for weight loss with morning workouts. I believe that morning workouts promote more caloric burn throughout the day. In the afternoon or evening our metabolic clock is already starting to slow down and we burn the least amount of calories towards the end of the day.

Is aerobic walking as healthy as jogging or running?

There are many factors that need to be established before someone chooses the exercises that they do on a regular basis. One of the most important aspects of fitness and health is that we need to maintain the health and safety of our joints. We need to find what type of muscular and anatomical dysfunctions we have and develop protocols that can either change these dysfunctions or choose exercises that do not contribute to joint injuries.

The exercises that we choose should be the safest for our individual bodies. If your body can run, especially in short burst intervals, without injuring itself, then this would be the best exercise for you, but for some people simply getting up from a seated position 10 times is a demanding, safe and an effective exercise.

Paul's company, IQ Fitness and Wellness, incorporates a comprehensive and holistic approach to weight loss, fitness, longevity and relief from chronic pain.

Paul can be reached at **iqpaul@gmail.com**

7 KIMBERLY WAGNER

What should people look out for when hiring a personal trainer?

The number one problem with choosing a trainer is most people don't even know where to begin! Don't be afraid to take this process slowly and do your research. More often than not we rush into a decision like this because we are so motivated to get started right now. Take time, ask questions, and be thorough in your search for better wellness.

Here are our top 10 questions you should ask when looking to hire a personal trainer:

1. Qualification/Education (Degree or Certification)?

Because personal training is not a monitored field, believe it or not, people can get their certification in one day online! Be certain that you are getting someone who has a nationally accredited certification or a Bachelors/Masters Degree in Exercise Science. At Impulse, we are extremely cautious with the certifications that we accept with our trainers. The only ones we currently accept are the American Council on Exercise (ACE), the National Academy of Sports Medicine (NASM), the National Strength & Conditioning Association (NSCA), the American College of Sports Medicine (ACSM), the National Exercise Trainers Association (NETA) and the National Federation of Professional Trainers (NFPT).

2. Experience?

Make sure to ask how many people with similar goals or medical conditions to you the trainer is currently working with or has previously worked with.

3. Insurance?

Ask your trainer to show you a copy of their liability insurance which will ensure that you are properly taken care of IF something were to happen during your session or as a result of it.

4. References/Results?

Feel free to ask your trainer if you could talk to someone who has worked with them. Written references are great, but talking to someone is often more informative. Also, ask about the results people have achieved with your particular goals or medical conditions. This is the way to make sure that your trainer is being honest with you and not just saying what you want to hear to get you to sign up.

5. Assessments?

An assessment is essential to know where your starting point is and to see how much progress you are making. Make sure to ask your trainer what is involved with the assessment. A basic assessment includes the following; height, weight, blood pressure, resting heart rate, body composition (optional), circumference measurements, upper & lower body flexibility, upper & lower body strength, core stability& strength and cardiovascular capacity.

6. Training Philosophy?

Every trainer has a unique style. To make sure that you are going to reach your goals and stick with them, ask your trainer what their sessions are like. If you dislike a certain exercise, such as running, make sure that your trainer doesn't have a belief that running is the only way to reach your goal. Have a trainer talk you through a typical workout and make sure that they are giving a workout that is applicable to you and not them.

7. What is your plan to help me?

Ask your trainer what their plan is to help you reach your goals and an expected timeline for getting there.

8. Outside Support?

When you train with a trainer you see them 1-5 hours a week so make sure that you are having some sort of support system in place for the other 163-167 hours each week.

9. Maintenance Stage?

Ask your trainer if they have a maintenance stage available that will provide you with additional options when you reach your goals.

10. Price/Packages/Payment options?

Package discounts should be available as should different payment options to fit most budgets. Often the most expensive way to pay is per session, but if you are not sure you want to commit, don't be afraid to pay per session until you know for sure.

You also want a trainer who will push you when you need it, but knows the proper way to do so. Some trainers will just get in your face, shout exercises at you and forget that it's their job to motivate you while encouraging you to reach new limits. It is great if you have a workout that leaves you huffing and puffing but when you get home, if they haven't given you the tools to be successful you will fail. The personality of a trainer is also something to take into consideration, because you will see that trainer between 1 and 5 times per week! If you can't stand them and dread going to your sessions because of a conflict in personality, then you will most likely not keep up your routine and will probably eventually ditch going to the gym altogether.

Always seek out gyms that have a firm mission statement that is driven by educating and motivating. This means two essential things: first, trainers are committed to continually educating and developing themselves so they are able to give you the best information currently available to help you reach your goals. Second, the trainers at these facilities should show that they do not fear your growth and eventual departure. Gyms that hire trainers that shout exercises survive only by keeping you as a dependent rather than an independent client who has the tools to reach any goal inside or outside the gym.

All of these are important when selecting a trainer. You want your sessions to be, well, "personal". They are your "personal" trainer because they fit you personally. Don't be afraid to ask a potential trainer questions or ask their mission or philosophy. Even ask about their training style before committing. When you find the right trainer you are more inclined to stay committed to your goals and training time. And that's what it's all about.

If someone has a friend who is in good shape who is willing to give them exercise advice, why is it still a good idea to hire a personal trainer?

We all know these fitness enthusiasts that have found something that works for them and they begin preaching about their way of getting to better health, but will it work for you? After working with clients for a long time, we have yet to find two clients that need the same workouts and need the same motivation techniques and have exactly the same goals. Everyone is an individual and should be treated that way. Let's say you are plagued with chronic pain in your knee and you have a friend with a killer body who participated in a high intensity boot camp. Does that mean the boot camp will be the best thing for you? Absolutely not. You need a less intense program that includes corrective exercises for your pain before you progress to a higher intensity program.

There is more to maintaining a healthy lifestyle than just a good workout. Nutrition, metabolic training, strength training, cardiovascular training, personal goals, limitations, abilities, and lifestyle must all be taken into consideration and combined in the proper way for a healthy lifestyle and for fitness goals to be attained.

Often friends have the best intentions and only want to help, but it is essential that you find a trainer who will look at your goals, your limitations, and your current wellness state and create a fitness program that is conducive to your lifestyle and will progress you to reach your goals. More often than not, listening to an unqualified friend will lead to injuries, frustration, and resentment!

Is it true that people should take periods of time off from working out? If so, how long should these "workout vacations" last and how frequently should they occur?

Rest is essential for muscle growth since training is simply breaking down your muscles and when you rest you are giving your muscles time to repair and grow. Different phases of training require differing amounts of rest. That is why creating a periodized training program can be more beneficial than simply doing all cardiovascular training or all strength training. In a periodized program you can continue to work different muscle fibers while resting the ones that previously worked. For instance, work your slow twitch (aerobic) muscles one day and the next day work your fast twitch (anaerobic) muscles. This gives your body time to

48

heal and grow those slow twitch muscles but allows you to continue working towards your goal and achieving it in a shorter period of time.

Here are some simple strategies to stick with: never do two consecutive days of complete upper or lower body resistance training; incorporate interval training into your cardiovascular program; if you participate in a high intensity full body workout, make sure you are properly hydrating yourself, and eating proper foods; leave yourself at least 1 day per week to completely rest from training so you can recover. Without proper nutrition and hydration you may need more days off because you are not giving yourself the adequate nourishment to rebuild those muscles.

This is why people who have a "clean" diet and drink plenty of water are able to work out harder and longer with a reduced risk of injury. When you don't give your body the fuel it needs and you work out hard the muscles will not rebuild as fast. You will continue to tear them down and often this results in a pull, or even worse, torn muscles.

What are some tips to help people stick with an exercise program and not quit?

Find your motivating factors, build on them, and create new habits. It is one thing to commit to an exercise program until you've reached your goal, but to continue on with the program after you've reached your goal is an entirely different thing.

Goal setting is essential and is one of the first things that all my clients do. There is a quote I love from Brian Tracy, author of Eat that Frog, "Goals are the fuel in the furnace of achievement." Keeping your goals specific, measurable, attainable, realistic, and timely will ensure that you not only know exactly where you are going, but know when you have arrived! Also, set mini-goals so that benchmarks can be reached and you can feel like you are making progress. Even small victories are victories and when you see that you are able to make changes for the positive for yourself you will be more inclined to stick with the program.

Find an accountability partner and allow them to keep you on the right track during tough times. We often have our clients email us or keep a journal during difficult times to make sure that they are making decisions that will help them reach their goals and not sabotage their efforts in the gym. A trainer may see a client between 1-5 hours a week but that leaves 163 or more hours to lose focus, so having someone you feel comfortable emailing, texting, or calling at any time is important. This can be someone you respect and admire, but avoid partnering with a spouse, family member, or close friend as most often this will backfire and cause feelings of resentment. There is nothing worse than being at a family reunion and having your spouse say, "Do you really think you should eat that!"

Often we base our motivation on how we will look instead of how we will feel. Are you tired of being tired and just want more energy or do you want to be able to play with your kids/grandkids? Then focus on those goals instead of focusing on weight loss. When the scale doesn't move it can be very discouraging, so focusing more on the fact that you have more energy and are more confident can be essential to keep you moving forward.

Place positive quotes and mantras in visible places. Getting clients to think positive from the moment their feet touch the ground in the morning makes a huge impact. You should never let your feet hit the ground before thanking God for a new day and saying one positive thing about the day you are about to begin.

Celebrate your successes with something that inspires you. Find one thing that truly makes you feel great. This can be a hobby, helping someone else, taking a "ME" day, a massage, etc., but typically we encourage avoiding using food as a prize because this can be sabotaging to your efforts. If you accomplish a goal, you should be proud of it and reward yourself by taking the time to recognize a job well done. This will also give you motivation to keep working towards the next goal.

What is a "drop set"?

Drop sets are a technique generally used for weight lifting and body building, but it can also be a great tool for getting an interval cardiovascular workout while strength training. The technique for drop sets is to continuously move through an exercise with a lower weight once the muscle "failure" has begun with a higher weight. You want to change weights quickly, so it is common to see drop sets performed on weight machines. However, it can still be done with free weights. This workout routine has been shown to build muscle strength and endurance, but should not be performed regularly. 2-3x/wk for one week out of a month is all that I recommend.

There is, however, much controversy over the duration they should be performed. Some say do it for a full week and work each muscle group, then continue with regular exercise after that. Others say no more than 2-3x/wk, once a month, and some even say even every other month.

An example would be a client performing a basic bicep curl. The person begins with the highest weight they can curl without compromising his/her form and begin doing the set. Once the arm became fatigued so much that the client could no longer lift without compromising his/her form she would immediately "drop down" in the set to a lighter weight, so if they began with 25lbs initially they may drop to 20 lbs. Then they continue the rep. Most professionals say to not exceed dropping down twice. So 25-20-15 reps total would be an example of a drop set with two drop downs.

If someone likes to listen to music on a personal music player with headphones when they work out, is this considered rude by most personal trainers?

Usually, when working with a trainer the gym will have music playing and if you have a good trainer they will be trying to educate you during your workout so you can be as informed as possible about your health and wellness. On several occasions we have worked with people who hold high stress jobs and just want to come in to the gym, and get away from the world for a while so they stick their headphones on and as long as they can hear instructions and follow the program without the trainer having to yell over the music it is fine. Every trainer is different and may have different guidelines, so if this is something that you are concerned about, bring it up before beginning with a trainer.

Which types of people can benefit the most from a personal trainer?

Anyone who is truly committed to making a change can benefit from a trainer. I don't believe that having a personal trainer is something that is reserved for the wealthy and those with ample free time. Personal training is about wanting more for yourself and identifying that you want the best way to make that happen.

Whether you need to get in shape, recover from an injury, or just stay fit a trainer can help. Even if you feel you are in shape, your body hits plateaus and a trainer can help you get over those or avoid them completely with a well-designed fitness program.

Look at personal training as the opportunity to further your education on how your life and your health are interrelated. If you want to educate yourself, you don't stop going to school, reading books, attending seminars or talking to professionals. You dig in, educate yourself and learn as much as possible. That is what a personal trainer should do for you: educate, motivate, and equip you to lead the healthiest lifestyle you can experience!

What are "boot camps" and why are they so popular?

Boot camps can be a variety of different styles of workouts depending on the trainer. They are typically a high intensity, interval style training that includes full body movements, minimal strength equipment, and anaerobic exercises. The main focus of most boot camps is to burn the maximum amount of calories in the shortest amount of time.

These metabolic style programs focus on caloric burn through functional training. That is, training that promotes a higher metabolism with movements that not only mimic everyday life but center on several large muscle groups at one time.

Boot camps have become wildly popular due to their efficiency and effectiveness. In a time crunched world it is next to impossible to get three 60 minute strength training days and four or more 45 minute cardiovascular sessions for the typical person. Boot camps allow you to not only get your heart rate up for an extended amount of time and build muscle, but also burn a ton of calories with only a couple of 45 minute sessions per week. There is also something fun and rewarding about going to a class with dozens of other people cheering you on and burning off those unwanted calories.

One last and very important thing, metabolic style training, which is what most boot camps are, also increases hormones that are responsible for lipolysis, or fat loss!

How can people overcome junk food cravings?

Identify what makes you crave the junk to begin with. Are you "comfort eating" because you are stressed or emotional? Is there something hormonal that is causing you to crave certain foods? And sometimes it actually is some medical condition. Cravings can be a sign of a deficiency. In fact, most people don't know that when they crave sugar it can mean a protein deficiency.

When you begin to have a craving be mindful and journal how you are feeling, and remind yourself of your long term goals. I love keeping a journal to write how I am feeling when those urges hit because more often than not they are brought on by something other than hunger. Stress, exhaustion, boredom, and many other emotions can give you the sensation that you need something sugary. But if you give in to a craving don't beat yourself up either. This is about learning how to work through obstacles and turning them into your greatest opportunity for change.

Most cravings pass after 10 minutes. So if you stop to think for a moment before you dive into the junk food, you are more inclined to decline the junk food. Also, "out of sight out of mind" is a common and true saying, so do it: get rid of the junk and surround yourself with healthy food. Then when you are having a craving you can't just jump into your cupboard and eat garbage.

Another great tip is to plan your meals so you don't have a chance to cheat. If you know exactly what you will be eating for that meal and it is ready to eat, it is much easier to say no to the cookie that's just sitting on the counter.

Eat things like grapefruit which is an appetite suppressant or a small handful of berries or sweet potatoes gives your body the sugar it is craving without ruining the diet. Veggies and dry seasonings on your chicken and fish help with the salt cravings. Almonds give a good crunch and are a healthy fat and protein. Pick healthy foods that trick your body into thinking it is getting those cravings fulfilled.

Do most personal trainers yell at people like drill sergeants to keep them motivated? What if someone wants to hire a personal trainer without being screamed at?

This goes back to knowing what your goals are and what you want in a trainer. If you carefully select the trainer you are working with, then you will weed out ones that do not fit your training style. Read testimonials, talk to people who you have seen working with the trainer, get feedback. We actually encourage new clients to come in and observe sessions before they commit to training so they can understand exactly what they are committing to and aren't shocked on the first day of training. Not every trainer screams. In fact, most use more proactive tools to motivate their clients.

How does someone know if they're "over-training"?

Over-training occurs when your physical state is affected because your body does not have adequate time to recover. This starts to cause pain and soreness and can lead to serious injuries such as ligament tears, strained muscles, and a wide ray of other injuries. Over-training can be aggravated by performing exercises that your body is not ready for. For instance, if you haven't exercised in a long time and you jump into a high intensity interval program that includes a lot of plyometric or jumping exercises, you are most definitely at risk for putting your body in a state of over-training very quickly. Training, like anything else, takes time and should be approached with a progressive program that begins slowly and gradually increases your intensity to avoid injury and over-training.

The best way to avoid over-training is listening to your body and observing the way it responds to certain exercises. Some will take longer to recover than others. If you feel your strength decrease and have no energy after a couple days of working out it is probably time to take a break and let your body heal.

Proper rest, hydration, and nutrition are also essential for recovery and avoiding injuries from over-training. Getting enough sleep, water, protein, carbohydrates, fats, nutrients, and vitamins into your body will allow your body to heal faster and stay injury free.

How will a trainer know what program is right for their client?

The trainer does initial assessments and meetings and learns about what the client's goals are, and then from there discusses their likes and dislikes when it comes to working out. All of the intake information helps to find programs that will motivate, encourage and ignite their client's passion for reaching his/her goals. Part of staying motivated comes down to how well a trainer can help create a program that is truly unique to the client and how the trainer and client adapt if, as the program progresses, it turns out to not be the correct fit. Never being afraid to adapt and change makes a good relationship, and helps to ensure proper programming is being utilized.

Is it typically acceptable for people to bring their children to a personal training session?

For the sake of the client and the trainer we strongly discourage bringing your kids to your session for numerous reasons. Often people commit to personal training as a chance to do something that is positive for them and if they feel like they are unable to concentrate on themselves during the session it can be frustrating. Also, for safety reasons we discourage having kids in the gym unattended. There are too many weights, balls, bands, etc. that can put the child at risk. The final reason we would discourage bringing children to a session is because you are paying a good price for a trainer and if they are running around babysitting instead of giving you the attention you are paying for it can be a waste of your money.

A few of our clients have adopted a trade system where one of them will babysit while the other works out and then switch on the other days. They love it because they can come to the gym and focus 100% on themselves!

If the child is old enough to participate and the client and trainer are ok with them jumping in on the session, this may be a great way to promote a healthy lifestyle to a young, impressionable child. Just make sure that the program is modified properly to avoid injuring the child.

How much sleep should people get when they exercise regularly?

Research shows that 8-10 hours of sleep is medically recommended for proper focus and function. There are numerous studies out there supporting the conclusion that lack of sleep not only affects your focus but also physical capabilities, cognitive functioning, and weight management!

When you are exercising regularly and tearing down your muscles you need to get adequate rest and sleep in order to recover and build your muscles properly. Lack of sleep can lead to increases in a hormone, cortisol, which inhibits the body's ability to repair tissue and cell damage done by exercise. Also, for those participating in extended periods of exercise (90 minutes or more) sleep deprivation can lead to a slower glycogen or energy storage. This will cause a person to operate on a much less than optimal level in their exercise routine.

Sleep has been directly linked to weight management issues due to the hormones that are released during the initial stages of deep sleep. These hormones (HGH in particular) are responsible for your body's fat and muscle storage. As we age we typically spend less time in a deep sleep and therefore our bodies emit less HG hormone. This is part of the reason weight management becomes more difficult with age. Feeling tired can also initiate cravings so when someone feels like they need that sugary snack it can be a sign that their body needs rest. This can lead to overeating, lethargy, and decrease your desire to exercise.

Is it customary for a personal trainer to provide references of satisfied clients?

Although it isn't customary for personal trainers to provide references of satisfied clients there is no harm in asking for references and it could be a great way to obtain valuable information and ensure that you are going to get the highest quality service.

Often it is difficult for a trainer to persuade a client to allow them to hand out the client's phone number but the trainer may have testimonials on paper, video, or even an email address where you can contact the client.

Another great way to obtain references is by asking to shadow a session and then talking with the client afterwards. This will give you a great idea of what goes on during a session as well as a chance to talk in person to a client who has been working with that trainer.

Feel free to contact Kimberly for further questions:
Email: kwagler@impulsetraining.com

Phone: 330-499-2266

Website: impulsetraining.com

Address: 7982 Whipple Ave NW

North Canton, OH 44720

8 CHRIS TERENZIO

Is it typical for a personal trainer to ask their clients to sign a contract? If so, what are some standard contract lengths and terms?

Many trainers do ask their clients to sign contracts. A contract adds legitimacy to the training process, can help the client with program adherence, and helps the trainer solidify income levels. Lengths and terms vary, but I have clients that commit to 30 sessions at a time (3 times a week for 10 weeks).

If someone also does yoga, should they work out on the same day that they have their yoga class?

Depending on the fitness level of the person and the goals that they are trying to achieve, yoga and strength training can be done on the same day. With that being said, I prefer to have my clients use yoga as an alternative form of exercise. This is something that I encourage them to do on days that they are not doing resistance training.

Is there a difference between "cardio" and "aerobic"? If there is, what's the difference?

Most people (as well as trainers) use the terms "cardio" and "aerobic" interchangeably. I think of "cardio" as exercise done primarily to improve the cardiovascular system (heart and lung function), while the main goal of "aerobic" exercise is to burn body fat. Of course, some "cardio" exercise can also help you burn fat and some "aerobic" exercise (when performed at the proper intensity) can improve heart and lung function. It's really just a technicality.

Can sit-ups help people lose belly fat? Why do some people do thousands of sit-ups and they still don't lose any belly fat?

Neither sit-ups, nor crunches, nor any other "abdominal" exercises can help you burn body fat. Body fat is burned off with intense resistance training, intense cardiovascular intervals and a sound nutritional plan. Sit-ups can help you tone the muscles of the abdominal region, but if you have a layer of excess body fat, you will never see those abdominal muscles.

What are some factors that impact a person's metabolism?

The factors that affect metabolism are: resistance training, the amount of lean body mass a person has, cardiovascular training, genetics and when, what and how much a person eats.

What can people do to stay motivated after they've started a workout program?

The best ways to stay motivated once you begin an exercise program are as follows: Hire a trainer to motivate you, find a training partner, join a class, train for a specific goal, and add as much variety to the workout as possible.

If someone enjoys drinking alcohol in moderation, how often can they indulge without feeling guilty or undoing all the progress they made with their trainer?

I believe that a couple of beers or a drink or two on the weekend is not going to have a major effect on a person's progress. If that person then extends this drinking to 2 or 3 nights per week things start to change. Monitor your body and how it is changing on a regular basis and remember the key word is "moderation."

If someone has a personal trainer do they also need a nutritionist? What are the differences between a personal trainer and a nutritionist?

A person who is working out with a personal trainer could also benefit from a nutritionist. While many trainers know enough about proper nutrition to make suggestions and to help you make better choices, they cannot create diets for their clients. Most trainers do not have the same level of education in nutrition as a nutritionist, and a trainer should not pass him or herself off as a nutritionist. Similarly, many nutritionists are in good shape, but they cannot train a client, as they do not have the same education as the trainer. They are two distinct areas of expertise, period.

What should people look out for when joining a gym?

When looking for a gym people should consider things such as: size (and how much equipment they have), price, classes offered, level of education of the trainers, cleanliness, clientele, staff friendliness, proximity to home, safety of parking lot. The potential member should also visit the gym at the time he or she would like to work out to see how crowded the facility is at that time.

When it comes to working out, there seems to be a lot of conflicting information out there. How can people know what advice is good and what is not?

The best way to get sound exercise advice is from an expert. In this case I mean a Personal Trainer who is certified by a reputable organization. A trainer with a degree in exercise science or a related field would be even better than one that is only certified. This trainer should have experience with a wide range of clients and should also be able to provide references.

How should someone's age be taken into consideration when starting a new exercise program?

Generally, as we age we tend to have more medical issues to take into consideration. However, there are ultra-fit people who are in their 50's, 60's, 70's and beyond. A full health history form should be completed by everyone and in most cases a physician's clearance should be given as well. Exercise tests can (and should) be administered to ensure the older client is able to handle an exercise program, and in many cases special care should be taken not to overwork joints such as knees and shoulders.

Does weight training cause people to lose flexibility?

Weight training does not cause people to lose flexibility. In fact, when weight training exercises are done through full and proper ranges of motion they can help improve a person's flexibility.

If someone can only work out once a week, should they even bother?

Even if you could only exercise once per week you should do it. I have a number of clients who only work out once per week, and they have made positive changes in their fitness level. It is very difficult to achieve optimal fitness exercising once per week, but every bit helps. Usually, people find that if they have the time and energy for one workout they can do another.

Other than losing weight and gaining muscle, what are some of the other benefits of getting in shape?

Getting in shape can help you prepare for an event (like a 5k run), or help you improve in a sport or activity (like golf, skiing or tennis). Working out also helps improve self-esteem, helps people sleep better, reduces stress, and gives them clarity of thought and increases energy levels.

What can people do if they "plateau" and stop seeing results from their workout routine?

If you hit a plateau, take a little break to reinvigorate your body. When you get back to the program you will have renewed energy. If that doesn't work, hire a trainer or take a class. As stated above, if you train with a goal or sport in mind, that should give you new focus. There are great manuals available for someone who is looking for a strength and conditioning program for a specific sport.

Chris Terenzio can be reached at In-Home Health & Fitness
58 Killian Avenue
Trumbull, CT 06611
Chris@bootcamp-ct.com
www.bootcamp-ct.com

9 CHARLENE REEVES

Exercise balls look unstable. Are they really safe?

Overweight and obese individuals should be cautious with exercise balls. Anyone can use an exercise ball as long as the ball is able to support their body weight and the exercises that they are performing are appropriate for their ability. Lower-end balls might only be able to support 250lbs, so it's best to find a good quality ball (sporting store or online) that can support well above your body weight. Some balls on the market can support 500+lbs and will last much longer than a lesser-quality ball. There are also burst-resistant balls that, if damaged, will slowly leak air as opposed to bursting rapidly.

I've heard that eating late at night causes weight gain. Is this true? Why or why not?

It's neither good nor bad to eat at any time of day. Eating should be based on hunger signals rather than time of day. If you feel hungry, your body is telling you that you need to eat to provide it with the fuel it needs to function properly. The criticism that eating at night has evoked is due to two factors. One, many people eat 50% or more of their calories for the day in the evening. Considering that if you are gaining weight you are eating more calories than your body needs, cutting back on calories consumed late in the day could help decrease your intake to a level that will maintain your weight or help you lose weight. Second, people tend to make unhealthy choices later at night, relying on snack foods rather than wholesome meals, while they watch TV or surf the internet.

How do I know if the weight I am lifting is too heavy?

First and foremost, if doing strength exercise, make sure you can control the weight you are using. If you cannot lift the weight without arching your back, leaning to one side or throwing it – it is too heavy and you need to lower the weight. Aside from this, abdominals should always be engaged (tight); shoulders back and usually all joints should be in alignment (knees, ankles, etc.). Head should also be in alignment with the spine.

Is a single workout better for weight loss than multiple workouts throughout the day?

In order to lose weight you must create a caloric deficit over time. You can do this by burning extra calories through activity and/or reducing your calorie intake. The American College of Sports Medicine recommends burning between 300 - 500 calories by physical activity on most days of the week. To lose weight they recommend a calorie deficit of 500 - 1000 calories per day. And because you create a calorie deficit across days, weeks and months, the actual number of calories you burn at once is inconsequential; therefore, it does not matter if you exercise in one session or several throughout your day.

Should someone who's trying to build muscle eat differently than someone who's looking to lose weight?

Usually those looking to build muscle eat more carbs and protein and tend to add supplements to their diet. Those looking to lose weight tend to eat less carbs, more fruits and vegetables while watching their caloric intake. Meet with a dietician to ensure you are eating the appropriate foods that will enable your success.

If I have to cancel an appointment with my trainer, will I be charged anyway?

Most gyms/trainers will have a cancellation policy that is clearly defined, and should be signed for by the participant, in their initial paperwork. Similar to a doctor, most trainers ask for anywhere between 12-24 hours' notice to cancel an appointment without penalty. Some gyms might offer one excused late cancellation and may be lenient with regard to weather, illness, or any other uncontrolled circumstances. When starting with a trainer, make sure you fully understand your gym/trainer's cancellation policy. If one is not printed and given to you in your initial paperwork, ask them to review the policy with you.

Is it okay to work out right after a meal?

How much you can eat and how close to a workout you can eat depends on the content of the meal, the intensity of the exercise, and to some degree, individual differences. Meals high in fat are slower to digest and can lead to gastrointestinal issues. High intensity exercise will cause more digestive problems than less intense exercise. Also, some people can simply tolerate food and liquid better before and during exercise than others. A basic guideline is to aim to eat 300 - 400 calories 1 - 2 hours before exercise. Most of those calories should be carbohydrates (whole grains, pasta and fruit are good examples), but the meal can also contain moderate protein (lean chicken, for example) and even a little fat (low-fat dairy is an example, but doesn't work for everyone). Experimenting with the total calories and the ratio of carbs, protein and fat is necessary to find what works for you.

If your timing is tighter, but you still need something to eat (for instance, you feel weak or lightheaded during your workouts), try cutting back on the portion size and don't worry if the meal is mostly carbohydrates. In fact, an easily digestible snack of about 15 g of carbohydrates, such as ½ of a medium banana, is great.

Note that 8 oz. of many energy drinks contain about 15g of carbohydrate. Therefore, if whole food is a problem, but you still feel like you need calories, this may be a good solution for you.

I'm not sure what to bring to my first session with my trainer. Any suggestions?

Bring a complete health history, a list of medications, and any other forms your trainer requires. Have a list of questions you might have for your trainer and a list of goals you want to accomplish. Aside from the paperwork, all you should bring is a commitment to your fitness goals! Of course, don't forget your best effort during that hour with your trainer – focus on each exercise and not other distractions. Most importantly, a bring a positive attitude.

How should people with medical conditions approach their workouts?

All types of people suffer from various medical conditions – pro athletes, weekend warriors, soccer players, swimmers, etc. People with a medical condition need to maintain a normal and healthy lifestyle too, and this includes exercise and other physical activities. People with a medical condition should follow their doctors prescribed medications, monitor symptoms and avoid triggers if possible. If they are having difficulty when exercising, they should talk to their doctor – many times small changes can be made that will provide relief and allow them to continue exercising.

How far ahead do I have to commit to when hiring a personal trainer?

Most clients prefer a specific day and time. We schedule sessions at the beginning of the month for that month to reserve their time slots. Each week we confirm the following week's scheduled appointments, in case there is a conflict. A small minority of clients prefer to schedule week to week. These clients only workout once a week with me and their availability varies. Clients that have a set time/day each week are more consistent and more successful with following an exercise program. It's a lifestyle choice for them and it's important for them to not miss their appointment.

It's hard for me to commit to a diet because there are foods I know I can't give up. What do you suggest?

The short answer is, don't give it up. There is no reason to give up a favorite food forever. And trying to give up a certain food forever can actually lead to "falling off the wagon" with your diet - often with your entire healthy diet, not just with the food in question. If you have a food that is such a powerful trigger for you that you cannot stop eating it, then do not keep it in the house. Give yourself permission to have it once in a while outside of your home as a special treat, such as going out for pizza or ice cream or having a soda with dinner in a restaurant.

How often should I work out my abs?

Like any muscle group, the abs will get overworked if exercised intensely every day. Many people who do physical jobs work the core muscles every day and have no problems. The answer can be tricky because it depends on what you mean by working your abs. Performing hundreds of crunches every day can cause postural imbalances which lead to upper back and neck problems. Balancing, flexion- extension and isometric core work can promote good posture and great abs. A trained yoga, Pilates personal trainer or physical therapist can teach you proper form and movements for these exercises. I recommend working the core muscles intensely every other day with your weight training program. If you combine that with cardiovascular exercise you will be burning fat more efficiently. Remember - spot reducing doesn't work.

Is it better for someone to work out at home or at a gym with their personal trainer? What are the pros and cons to each?

This question has no absolute answer. What fits your personality and where will you be most focused?

The gym provides a variety of equipment, social interaction, support and a sense of community. There is also the aspect of motivation by working out with others. Gyms are less expensive than a trainer coming to your home. Gyms also provide an escape from home, school or work and the distractions that come from each.

Home provides a lower intimidation factor, increased privacy and solitude, less outside distraction, but often more internal distractions (kids, laundry, phones, etc.). Obviously, working out at home means no travel time.

The real question is what environment will best motivate and support you?

Charlene Reeves can be reached at TRAINING PARTNERS INC. – 863 Merrimon Avenue, Asheville, NC 28804 – 828-252-0920.

10 PATRICIA FAY

If someone just recently had surgery, can they lift weights or work out? What should be taken into consideration in these situations?

Since there are a wide variety of possible surgical procedures, it's best to speak with your physician about what you can expect immediately following your surgery. Their guidelines should be strictly adhered to, despite the fact that the patient might be feeling fine. It is best to inform your doctor of the details of your current workout program. If you do this and ask them specific questions, they will be able to advise you more accurately. For example, a patient may be able to resume a modified walking program soon after surgery, but will be cautioned about weight lifting for a few weeks. After receiving instructions from the doctor, the patient would then communicate them to their trainer or physical therapist.

Is it possible to lose fat and gain muscle at the same time? If so, how can this be done effectively?

Yes, this is possible, especially for someone who is just beginning an exercise regimen. It is sometimes referred to as "recompositioning". If someone has been inactive and they begin an exercise program their body will need to create more muscle to perform the additional workload. To best add muscle, a mixed program of cardiovascular and resistance training is beneficial. Weight training, also called resistance training will cause your body to increase the size of the existing muscle fibers as well as add new ones. You may also need more muscle fibers to complete the cardio you choose. Generally however, resistance training is considered a building type of exercise while cardio is used for fat burning. To lose body fat one needs to consume fewer calories than needed, thus creating a caloric deficit. A complete program for building muscle and burning fat would include both types of exercise mentioned above along with a calorie-controlled eating plan and adequate rest and sleep.

If someone has been a "yo-yo dieter" their entire lives, how can a personal trainer help a person them?

That's a great question. It's important to address what is within the scope of practice of a personal trainer and what is not. Unless a trainer has specific nutrition training they are not qualified to make nutritional recommendations. However, through a well-designed program of exercise they can help someone improve their health and achieve the goal of weight management. Exercise produces a wealth of beneficial changes in the body and mind which can reinforce positive behaviors like good eating choices. If the client sees they can maintain and even lose weight with exercise they may be more apt to stick to healthier behaviors. The trainer may also model what a healthy lifestyle is for the client so they can see how attainable it actually is.

What is the difference between a "high impact" and a "low impact" workout?

Generally speaking, a high impact exercise places more psi (pounds per square inch) on the foot than a low impact exercise. During a high impact exercise you may have both feet off the ground at the same time vs. one foot being on the floor at all times during low impact. Examples of this would be trail running versus a low impact step class.

How much of a say should the client have in determining which exercises they do?

It is always beneficial for the client to have input. It is helpful to have the client explain their likes and dislikes to the trainer. The program will have limited success if the client is run through exercises they do not like or feel they don't do very well. For long term adherence the client needs to enjoy the exercises chosen. They also need to see progress with their strength and conditioning too. The job of the trainer is to create a program that mixes familiar with unfamiliar exercises, instruct the client how to achieve proper intensity and form, mix things up to keep it fresh, and to assure progress is being made.

Why do certain "non-fat" foods still make people gain weight?

Simply put, because over consumption of any food can result in adding fat to your body. If you eat more than you need you will gain fat whether it comes from low-fat, non-fat or low-sugar foods.

Is it true that some exercises produce results faster than others? Is so, which exercises provide the best and worst "return on investment"?

It's important to know what result you are going for. If you wanted to put on 10 lbs. of muscle, endless miles of running would not result in that goal. If you wanted to drop 20 lbs. of fat, hours of yoga might not be the best way to go. All properly prescribed exercise is beneficial, but you need to first identify what your goals are and then choose the best type of exercise for meeting that goal. If you want to add that 10 lbs. of muscle, you would spend a great part of your time in the gym doing various types of resistance training. If your goal is to increase aerobic conditioning, you would spend more time doing interval training on cardio machines or working on cardio outdoors.

I feel the best exercises combine lots of elements. I like exercise to be functional and incorporate resistance training and cardio at the same time. I also like for them to utilize upper, lower and core sections of the body. These exercises that use all muscle groups in a functional way are also great calorie burners. One example might be picking a dumbbell up from the floor on the outside of your left foot and visualizing placing it up on a high shelf above your head near the outside of your right arm. This uses your whole body and mimics something you would do in life.

How should someone determine how many grams of protein and carbs they should be eating each day?

There are many resources on-line and good books to read today. It obviously depends on the individual person's lifestyle and goals. A couch potato will have very different needs than a professional athlete. The only real answer here is to consult with a Registered Dietitian or RD.

Is it a good idea for someone to work out if they have a cold?

It depends on the severity of their symptoms. Exercise can suppress the immune system in the short term even though over the long term it improves it. If you are feeling fatigued and compromised, the last thing you need would be exercise. You may need to rest instead. I have also read that some people create a line at the neck. If the cold is above that line or a head cold, exercise is a "yes". If it is localized to the lungs, it's best to wait. I think it's important to know how long someone has been sick. If it's within the first couple of days, I would generally advise against it, but if it's at the tail-end, they should be fine. I would also avoid the gym if I were contagious.

Is it better to perform cardio before or after lifting weights, or should cardio be done on a completely different day?

If you are going to combine the two, I recommend weights first. Weight training is about intensity and having all the strength you can muster. If you deplete your energy with cardio before you have even begun, your weight session will suffer. If your goal is fat loss, research suggests that by the time you have used up energy lifting weights and then move onto cardio you may be burning more fat for fuel.

I do like to separate them out but if someone has limited time they can be done together on the same day. If you base your eating on your exercise schedule you may want to eat differently pre- and post-exercise for cardio and weights. For this reason it makes sense to do them on different days.

Is it better to exercise every part of the body on the same day, or is it better to focus on different muscle groups on different days? Please explain why one is better than the other.

This topic has been researched extensively. One study showed that a whole body routine with one set of 12 reps for one exercise per body part produced the same or near to the same results as a split routine which works fewer body parts in a day. I generally start a client on total body workouts every other day. If they have the ability to get to the gym almost every day and have more experience it behooves someone to break the body parts up. That means you have more work for each muscle and they get longer rest periods between training.

If someone doesn't have the time to spend hours cooking healthy meals, how can they still eat healthy?

There are many options. Healthy food doesn't have to be complicated. Actually, it's quite the opposite. How many body builders do you see building complex sauces and fussing with the look of each plate? Healthy food is simple food - oatmeal, chicken breasts, steamed veggies, fruit, etc. I generally cook twice a week; Wednesday and Sunday when I have more free time. I make 6-9 chicken breasts, quinoa, a big pot of oatmeal, and other healthy choices. You can even make all the components of a healthy meal like chicken, brown rice and veg and freeze it in a freezer-safe plastic container for your own frozen dinner! Products like protein powders make it easy and quick to get a high quality protein source for your daily intake.

What should a personal trainer take into consideration when working with each individual client?

They should start with a conversation to see if their personalities match. After that they need health history, exercise history, likes and dislikes, and so on. The client's needs are of the utmost importance. It is the trainer's responsibility to assess whether or not they are qualified to work with a client. Many times prospective clients do not ask about education or certification. Most clients know what they want to achieve, but don't ask the trainer to explain how their work experience might benefit that client. I have seen trainers take on any client whether they have the knowledge to adequately serve that person or not.

If someone isn't sore after a workout, does that mean they didn't work out hard enough?

No, that's not true. While some people may use this as a yardstick for measuring success of the previous workout, lack of soreness does not always indicate lack of progress. A newbie will be sore from almost anything they do while a seasoned exerciser will most likely have less soreness after a workout. The experienced exerciser should periodically switch up their routines though to make sure they are progressing. When they switch it up they should feel some new soreness.

The new fad seems to be "buying organic". Is there any validity to eating organic food over non-organic food? What are the benefits and/or things to be aware of?

I think it's valid. First, it's kinder to the planet to have less pesticides used. Second, the nutrition may or may not be improved, but I think everyone can agree the fewer pesticides and chemicals we ingest the better. Organics can be expensive so I use one rule. If I intend to eat the skin I buy organic. If it something I intend to peel like a navel orange I might be able to save some money by buying non-organic oranges. If you can afford to buy organic food, I say go for it.

Be aware that even though certain companies are liberal with their product labeling, some products cannot truly be called organic. One such example is fish. If they circulate in the ocean and ingest contaminants from around the world, I wouldn't call that organic. They may be fed strictly organic food pellets but they are also ingesting what's available in the seas.

Patricia can be reached via telephone or internet.

Patricia@beyondexpectationscoaching.com

Her website is www.beyondexpectationscoaching.com

802/310-2378

11 BRYAN J. PETTIT

Does it make a difference if someone just does all of their exercise over the weekend instead of spreading it out over the week?

No. I have many corporate executives that I work out with that are on the road for business during the week and because of packed schedules, they only have time to get workouts in on the weekends. My recommendation is to get a weekday workout in to go with a Saturday and Sunday workout, even if it means buying some dumbbells for their home to just get a couple of exercises in before bedtime or right after work.

How often should someone workout with a personal trainer?

I would recommend 2 to 3 times per week to start with. Most clients begin using a personal trainer because they are trying to incorporate a new "healthy lifestyle." By working with a personal trainer 2 to 3 times per week for 6 to 12 weeks at a minimum, they are more likely to succeed in making working out a pattern in their weekly schedule.

Is coffee bad for someone who is trying to lose weight or get in shape?

Not necessarily. Regular coffee really does not have many calories in it. However, many of the "coffee mixes" that one will buy from coffee shops are loaded with calories. These drinks will hinder a client's results dramatically, since some of these drinks have as many as 1,000 calories in them. I usually recommend certain herbal teas to my clients that will give them a caffeine source, but also antioxidants which coffee doesn't supply.

How can a personal trainer help a client with nutrition?

When I have a new client, I give them a "goal specific" nutrition program to follow. This plan offers fast and easy options that take the "I don't have time" excuse out of eating healthy. If a client still feels this has not helped them, then we sit down and rework the nutrition program to make it as quick, easy, and realistic as possible.

Is it unhealthy to eat a vegetarian or vegan diet that has no meat or dairy?

No. I have several vegan clients that I have worked with and they have seen as great results as my non-vegan clients. With the high quality supplement products on the market today, vegetarians can still achieve their protein goals without having to eat an abundance of calories.

Once someone begins working out with a personal trainer, what goes on during the sessions?

Each client is different, based on their goals and sessions they have agreed to. Most train for a 60 minute period and do a combination of weight training, balance training and core training. I prefer that clients do cardio on their own and I try to make sessions fast paced enough for my weight loss clients to receive cardiovascular benefits from the session.

How long should a personal training session last?

No more than 60 minutes. If anyone spends more than 60 minutes in the gym they are not working hard enough.

How much will it cost to hire a personal trainer?

Working at the gyms, I would see specials run as low as $33 per session and I have people pay as much as $100 per session for prime times during the day. One should be willing to pay a little more to hire a trainer with an exercise or human performance degree. Be sure that certifications are posted, because, in my experience, many gyms are more worried about customers making them money than qualifications of their trainers, which means they will undercut the personal trainer industry all the time.

Is it better to work out for a long period of time at a low intensity or a short period of time at a high intensity?

This depends on the person's workout experience. Any workout that is not at least 30 minutes long, will not allow a person to get the full cardiovascular benefit from the workout. So, if someone is crunched for time, I would recommend a 30 minute workout at the highest intensity they can perform.

How do people get rid of loose skin after weight loss?

For the loose skin that does not snap back within a year after losing significant amounts of weight, the only option is "lift" surgery. I have had clients that have lost 100 pounds or more that have had to have tummy tuck, breast lift and butt lift surgeries done because they are not happy with loose and sagging skin after a significant weight loss.

How do people measure their heart rate?

Because of the low cost devices available, many people use watches and bands to measure their heart rate. If I have a client that does not have either, then I will check their heart rate either manually or by grabbing the heart rate foils on the treadmill.

Why is it that, no matter how much cardio some people do, they still can't lose weight?

I find that most people who tell me they are doing cardio "all the time" are either performing low-to-no intensity cardio or dramatically cheating on their nutrition plan. By consuming more calories than they burn, they will never lose weight.

Do men lose weight faster than women?

No. Many people have this perception because a women's ideal weight is so much less than a man's. Because it takes more calories to maintain a higher weight, the more a male client cuts back their food intake, the quicker they achieve their ideal weight, which leads many of their female counterparts to believe the male lost weight faster.

Is there an ideal time of day to work out?

No. I have seen studies that have claimed morning or afternoon to be better, but actually working with clients has proved to me that each person's body responds differently to the time of day they are working out, so it is up to each individual to determine what time of day works best for them.

Is aerobic walking as healthy as jogging or running?

If someone is doing "aerobic walking" it should be because they are incapable of running or jogging due to medical reasons. A client's heart rate will not get as high walking as jogging or running, which means they will not get the cardiovascular benefits they would get from running or jogging. Starting out, I have many of my clients jog for 30 - 60 second intervals and then walk for 1 - 2 minutes, until they are able to jog or run for at least 30 minutes straight.

Bryan J. Pettit can be reached at

Golden Trainer Performance Studio, Inc.
1066 Center Point RD NE
Cedar Rapids, Iowa 52402
319-721-4922
bpettit@goldentrainer.com

12 BOB FIELDS

Is it better to lift weights with free weights or with weight machines?

The correct answer to this question is, "it depends…" There are pros and cons to both types of training. The benefits of machines are that the movements are restricted to a fixed path or trajectory, while free weights provide multiple degrees of freedom, thus recruiting additional muscle and providing the best range of motion. If you're new to exercise and unsure of how to perform the exercises correctly and/or have a pre-existing injury, you're better off sticking with machines. The starting and ending range of motion can be better controlled using machine technology as opposed to free weights. If you are a seasoned exerciser, then free weights would provide a better range of motion along with recruitment of additional muscles.

Why is one better than the other?

In my opinion, one isn't better than the other. It totally depends on the initial goal of the exercise participant. I've been a personal trainer for over 36 years and I've seen excellent results using both disciplines. If the participant's goals are not of a sport specific nature or one of figure/bodybuilding, then both disciplines can be used interchangeably, providing a nice variety, thereby, better confusing the muscles, which is what's really important to prevent plateauing or acclamation.

Is it true that eating too many vegetables will make most people gain water weight?

That would depend on many factors, e.g., what type of vegetables, how much sodium is contained in the vegetables, if the person is even susceptible to water retention due to sodium, food allergies and sensitivities, and pre-existing genetic conditions. For the most part, the average person experiences slight water retention due to any carbohydrate ingestion, and the amount of retention is specific to each person.

Can someone do resistance training if they don't own weights or belong to a gym?

Most definitely! There are many ways to do resistance training without the use of any equipment at all. Strength training is accomplished simply by targeting one or more muscle groups and applying resistance across a particular range of motion and repetitions. Typically, the average non sport specific exerciser would select an intensity or weight resistance such that the number of repetitions to achieve muscle fatigue or failure would fall between 8 and 15 reps. This can easily be accomplished by many methods. For example, if a person does straight leg push-ups and can only do 15 or so repetitions, then there is no difference between this mode and say, a seated chest press machine with a weight setting that produces the same result. A very popular mode of exercise nowadays is called "boot camp".
This form of exercise incorporates many movements which rely on gravity and one's own body weight to accomplish strength training. Additionally, there are many other methods and techniques which provide excellent resistive training, some of which include the use of elastic tubing, kettle bells, suspended ropes and/or cables, etc. The bottom line is to choose an activity or mode that provides the appropriate resistance given the current exercisers level of fitness.

Do people really lose muscle as they get older?

The answer is yes, however it's not muscle we lose its muscle *mass*. The number of muscle fibers remains the same, it's the cross-sectional size and the number of recruited fibers that diminish over time.

If so, how much muscle do they lose on average, and can anything be done to slow down this process?

The typical rule of thumb is that we lose an average of 5% of our muscle mass every 10 years after the age of 35. This has a lot to do with diminishing growth hormone, testosterone levels and sedentary lifestyle. Many individuals who continue to strength training in their adult life can maintain or even increase muscle mass.

How can someone figure out how many calories they should be eating each day?

There are many formulas available to do this. The best way, however, is to calculate your BMR, or basal metabolic rate first. Once this is done, you simply add a multiplier based on activity levels. For example, if you are sedentary with little or no exercise, multiply your BMR times 1.2. If you do moderate to light exercise 1 to 3 days a week, multiply your BMR times 1.375. If you're moderately active 3 to 5 days per week, multiply your BMR times 1.55. If you're very active and exercise between 6 and 7 days a week, then multiply your BMR times 1.725. And finally, if you train extra hard every day, multiply your BMR times 1.9. Note that these are rough estimates and are used to calculate the amount of calories to maintain current body weight, not necessarily to lose or gain. To lose or gain weight adjust your calories up or down accordingly.

Is it true that muscle will turn to fat if someone stops working out?

Absolutely false! Muscle and fat are two distinct types of tissues. Over time, with lack of use, the muscle will diminish in size, which we call atrophy, and will get weaker. Typically, a person's workouts diminish while their caloric intake remains the same. Thus, they gain fat on top of a muscle which is experiencing atrophy. To an uneducated observer, it appears as if muscle is turning to fat.

What is "body fat percentage"?

Body fat percentage, also sometimes called body composition, is simply the ratio of a person's fat divided by the person's total weight times 100.

How does this differ from "body mass index"?

Body mass index (BMI) is a rough estimation of a person's level of fat based on weight and height. It is adequate for the average sedentary population, but when used on athletes it produces erroneous results and is, therefore, not the preferred method of measurement. I personally don't use BMI at all in my business. Even at the local bariatric hospital where I work, we calculate BMI, but then still take a very accurate percent body fat measurement, which provides more useful and accurate information.

What can thin people do to build muscle?

Thin people, sometimes referred to as ectomorph body types, typically require more frequent workouts while supplementing with increased caloric intake. Unlike the average population, if they stop working out on a regular basis, they actually lose weight while the rest of us would gain.

Can couples or groups of people work out with a personal trainer at the same time?

Most definitely yes! This is very popular among trainers whose clients can't afford an exclusive one-on-one personal trainer. It's actually a win-win for both the trainer and the clients. Typical group training numbers are between 2 and 4 participants. More participants than that…we will just call that a boot camp.

If someone hasn't worked out in years, how should they get started in the safest way possible?

The safest way possible would include a visit to their doctor to acquire what is called a physician's release to exercise. Once this is obtained, they should think about what they want to accomplish and during what time frame. For the average person, wanting weight loss and to regain some strength, this would typically include some cardiovascular exercise combined with strength training 2 to 3 times a week. Regardless of their game plan, anything they do or start back doing, should be done at low to medium levels of intensity with a gradual progression across several weeks so as not to traumatize the body or cause injury.

Is it safe to work out first thing in the morning on an empty stomach?

Working out first thing in the morning is fine. However, I do not recommend it on an empty stomach. The human body requires blood sugar to function and after sleeping all night, blood sugar is usually pretty low. Almost all of my clients perform better and are much stronger after having eaten something for breakfast. As a matter of fact, when a client performs poorly, I usually ask them, "What were you thinking skipping breakfast?"

Do personal trainers usually have insurance?

Typically, the better, more experienced trainers do. Nowadays, it's difficult for a certified personal trainer to find work in the gym or health club without first proving or supplying proof of liability insurance.

How can people with very busy work schedules and family commitments fit working out into their schedule?

They make time! I know... easier said than done. My typical guilt trip speech includes the difference between "have to" and "should" in your life. You go to work every day because you have to. You schedule appointments and show up for them. Why? Because you have to. Unfortunately, for most people, exercise is a "should" and gets put off or displaced by the "have to" activities. To truly integrate exercise into one's life, it must become a "have to". Also, people find a way to carve out time for things that are truly important! My clients just assume that because I'm a trainer, I must work out every day for hours. The fact of the matter is that after training between 5 locations, the hospital and my in-home clients, I have very little time left over for my own workouts. My solution? I treat myself the way I would any client full of excuses. I used the only remaining time available to me. This meant purchasing an in-home piece of equipment and doing my own workouts at night after dinner. Where there's a will there's a way!

How many grams of fat should people consume each day, if they want to lose weight?

That's totally dependent on the person's initial weight and whether or not he or she has medical issues such as hypoglycemia or diabetes. A rule of thumb is no more than 30 gm. a day for female and 45 gm. for a male. But this would be for the average size population. Adjustments must be made for the morbidly obese. Too little fat can be bad also.

What are some of the most common myths about building muscle?

There are many myths when it comes to building muscle. One of my favorites is that you need tons of protein to create muscle. The fact of matter is adequate sources of protein and proper hydration are all you need. The secret is overloading the muscle properly during a workout. Another myth is that to achieve ideal muscle development you must do 10 to 12 repetitions. The fact of the matter is variety is key. Vary your workouts! For a few weeks try 15 to 22 reps followed by a few weeks of 6 to 8 followed by a few weeks of 10 to 12. You'll find that by confusing the muscles you prevent plateauing, promoting more efficient muscle growth.

You can contact Bob Fields at
Precision Health & Wellness
484 E. Carmel Dr. #186
Carmel, IN 46032
(317) 502-7570
E-Mail: trainerbob@precisionhealthandwellness.com
Web site: http://www.precisionhealthandwellness.com

13. GINA PAULHUS

Should people wait until they're not sore from their previous workout to start working out again?

It is not necessary to wait until soreness dissipates to work out again. However, it is best to avoid resistance training or strength training for the same muscle group two days in a row. For example, if you work your chest and triceps using a bench press on Monday, do not perform this same exercise on Tuesday. However, you may perform squats, which work the legs and glutes, on Tuesday.

It is also best to avoid performing high intensity exercise more than four days per week. For example, sprint work, interval training where you exercise to exhaustion for a minute at a time with a break in between, or weight lifting are all considered high intensity and should not be performed more than four days per week. However, jogging, yoga, and other lower intensity efforts may be performed up to six days per week.

If you experience excessive soreness on a daily basis, you are probably doing too much for your recovery capacities, and you will not enjoy the same fitness gains as the body gets stronger during rest, not during the actual workout. However, occasionally working out while sore will do you no harm.

Soreness is also not always an indicator of how hard you worked. It's possible to have a great workout and not feel sore. You are also much more likely to be sore when the exercise is one you have never done or have not done in a while. You are also more likely to be sore from exercises with an eccentric component where your muscles have to 'break' against gravity such as with plyometrics (jumping exercises). Soreness is genetic as well and some individuals experience more soreness than others.

If someone reaches their fitness goals, should they still continue to work with a personal trainer?

If someone reaches their fitness goals, it is still helpful to keep in touch with a personal trainer. Meeting once a month, once every three months, or even once every six months helps keep the client accountable to maintain the good results. It also provides an opportunity for the trainer to modify the exercise routines since the body adapts to the same routine done over and over. Also, boredom can set in if the routines are not changed up periodically. Finally, little injuries and other concerns can crop up from time to time and it's good to be able to run any concerns by the trainer. If you are no longer able to work with a trainer, try to find an exercise buddy to help keep you accountable, and subscribe to some fitness magazines or buy some books or DVDs for new ideas to keep your workouts fresh.

When people first start exercising, why do they sometimes gain weight initially?

When people first start exercising, the body undergoes some changes that can cause an increase on the scale. The first change is that an active body that is exercising regularly begins to store more carbohydrates in the muscles. Carbohydrate storage requires extra water storage in the muscle, and this shows up as a pound or two weight gain on the scale (this weight will be lost if you stop exercising, and is 'water' weight not fat weight). Also, when working out, some muscle building and fat loss are happening at the same time. In the beginning, muscle is built faster than fat is lost, and this may shows up as a (temporary) gain on the scale. Over time muscle building will slow down but fat burning will continue, and the scale will eventually go down as long as your diet is on point.

If someone has a heart condition, can they still work out?

In most cases, those with a heart concern are able to work out, and in fact, working out is helpful for the vast majority of those with a heart concern to help manage their condition. However, it is crucial to receive a physician's go-ahead before engaging in an exercise program if you have a heart concern. In general, working out is the best thing you can do for your heart. Inform your doctor if you have a heart concern and wish to begin an exercise program, especially if you take medications, because exercise can affect the dosages you may need and the timing of your dosages.

If someone has a job where they don't move around a lot, what can they do to increase their activity during the day, when

they're not working out?

If someone has a sedentary job, it is very important to move around for at least 5 minutes every hour. Every hour you sit, try to spend 5 minutes performing stretches by your desk, or 5 minutes walking around the office. If you have a colleague you need to communicate with, take a walk to chat with him or her rather than sending an email. Take a few extra laps when making a trip to the bathroom. If you work from home, stand up every hour and do a few quick chores rather than sit at your desk hour after hour. The increase in circulation and change of scenery will do wonders for your focus and concentration, and you will get much more done when you return to your work. Furthermore, when sitting for hours on end, your body is more inclined to lose muscle mass and increase fat mass. Lastly, sitting and doing repetitive work hour after hour can lead to overuse injuries such as carpel tunnel, and you will be more likely to prevent this if you take little breaks.

Is it safe for pregnant women to work out?

It is generally safe for pregnant women to work out, as long as the workout is not something new they were not performing before getting pregnant. It is always important to get your doctor's approval while pregnant before exercising, and to keep in touch with your doctor as your pregnancy progresses.

The biggest concern when exercising while pregnant is overheating. Great care must be taken to avoid overheating. This may require taking frequent breaks while exercising. You will need lots of fluids, cool clothing and a fan. It is important not to let the heart rate rise above 145 beats per minute while pregnant. The joints become more lax during pregnancy, so avoid movements that require large ranges of motion, such as chest flys or squats.

As the pregnancy progresses, avoid exercises which involve lying on the back, or pressing against the stomach (such as chest-supported rows). Also avoid overhead movements, as they can cause blood pressure to spike. Avoid exercises that require a strong grip for the same reason (such as strenuous bench-pressing or dumbbell chest-pressing). Never hold your breath during exercise. You may find that you need to modify or eliminate exercises which involve excessive head movement, such as stiff-legged deadlifts, as they may cause nausea or dizziness in a pregnant woman. Avoid prolonged periods of standing. Balance will eventually be a concern, so in the second and third trimester, reduce and eventually eliminate the Olympic lifts and perform demanding overhead lifts while seated. One of the most typical problems encountered by pregnant women is back pain. Their center of gravity shifts because extra weight is added over the nine months. Women tend to slouch the shoulders and arch the lower back to compensate for these changes, which of course leads to discomfort. A strong abdominal column as well as a strong back gained through weight training exercises before pregnancy can alleviate much of this problem, so assistance work geared to this need is helpful. Bodyweight exercises, such as unweighted lunges, present a useful alternative as the pregnancy develops, as do exercises which take some weight off the joints, such as swimming or cycling.

If someone prefers to work out without a personal trainer, can a trainer still help them get started? How would this work?

Most trainers are able to offer a 'jump-start' program which will help you develop an exercise routine that is customized for your body and goals, with the intent that you will be able to perform the routine on your own once you've learned it. Beware of trainers who only offer six-month or year-long contracts. There is no reason you cannot receive instruction and then work on your own, especially if you are familiar with correct form and body mechanics, and have no injuries.

Can someone use a personal trainer to help them rehabilitate from a sports injury? How would this be handled?

Some trainers are able to work with individuals who need rehabilitation. Ideally a client who needs injury rehabilitation begins with a physical therapist, but due to insurance many patients are discharged from therapy before they are recovered enough to jump back into their sport at full tilt. This is where a trainer can come in handy. Make sure the trainer you hire to help with sports injury rehabilitation has experience and expertise in the area of concern. Not all trainers are educated in this area.

When it comes to nutrition, it seems that few experts can agree on what is a healthy diet and what is not. How can people know which advice to take, with all of the contradictory information out there?

It is best to work with a certified nutritionist, preferably a sports nutrition specialist (even if your only 'sport' is exercise in the gym) when there are nutrition concerns. When in doubt, always go back to basics: beware of anyone who tells you to completely avoid entire food groups or macronutrients (the macronutrients are fat, carbohydrates and protein). A healthy, balanced diet doesn't exclude groups of foods, but rather includes a balance and variety of healthful nutritious foods, with room here and there for the occasional splurge. Beware of 'diets' that claim you can lose more than 2 lbs. per week. Unless you are morbidly obese, it is unhealthy to lose more than 2 lbs. per week, and if you do, the weight loss is water and lean tissue, not the fat mass you really need to lose.

If a personal trainer is always showing up late, should the client still be expected to pay for the full session? What's the customary way to deal with a situation like this?

If a personal trainer is always showing up late, at the very least the session should still last for the agreed upon length of time. If it starts ten minutes late and was scheduled for an hour, the client should still receive an hour of instruction. Traveling trainers deal with traffic and other clients running overtime due to special issues that may have come up. However, habitual tardiness is unprofessional and is a big red flag. If you address the concern with the trainer and the situation continues, start shopping for a trainer who is more respectful of your time.

Is it a good idea to eat any specific foods immediately before or after exercising?

It is important to consume a meal or snack that contains at least 25 grams of carbohydrates and 15 grams of protein either before or after exercising, but not both. If you have a regular meal before or after exercise, that is sufficient. It is not necessary to consume special shakes or bars before or after exercise - however, many people find a protein shake or bar to be a convenient way to get these nutrients. If you eat right before the exercise session, the nutrients will be available to your body as the exercise occurs and will still be in your system as your body recovers after the exercise session is over. However, as long as you consume the food right after exercise, your body will recover well and some prefer exercising on an empty stomach to avoid nausea. Whichever feels best to you is fine. If you do not take any food before or after exercise, your body will fail to recover as quickly or completely from the exercise and you will tend to burn off muscle rather than fat when you exercise. It's also very important to consume plenty of fluids before, during, and after exercise, and in most cases plain water is just fine. Sports drinks tend to include excess sugar which is not needed and will hinder the fat burning effects of the workout.

Should people with low blood sugar do anything differently before, during, or after a workout?

People with low blood sugar should take care not to exercise on an empty stomach. Furthermore, the overall diet should be catered to address the hypoglycemia (low blood sugar). This webpage explains the proper diet for those with hypoglycemia: http://www.umm.edu/altmed/articles/hypoglycemia000090.htm

Always check with your doctor before beginning an exercise program if you suffer from hypoglycemia. While exercising, always have a snack on hand you can use if your blood sugar dips, and start with short, easy exercise sessions until you are familiar with how your body responds to the exercise.

Is it true that it's bad to eat too much fruit because of all of the sugar it contains?

Too much of any one type of food is a bad idea, but it is difficult to consume too much sugar through fruit alone. Fruit contains natural sugar which is not as harmful to your body as processed sugar. It is also packed with fluids, fiber and vitamins and minerals, all of which make fruit worthwhile to consume. It is recommended you consume 5 to 9 servings of fruits and vegetables per day, and approximately half of those servings can come from fruits and half from vegetables. If you are interested in weight loss, try to choose more vegetables to round out your 5 to 9 servings. The less processed the fruit the better--for example, a fresh apple is better than applesauce, applesauce is better than 100% apple juice, and juice that is less than 100% juice is next to worthless. Processed fruit is stripped of nutrition and contains more sugar than unprocessed fruit. Dried fruits, although healthy, are easy to over consume because almost all of the water is removed. If you need to lose weight, try to avoid dried fruits or make sure you measure the portion size. Just a quarter cup is typically one serving.

How accurate are the calorie counters on gym machines?

The calorie readout on cardio machines are not reliable. Treadmills and rowing machines tend to be the most accurate, followed by bikes and step mills (the revolving staircase machine). Elliptical trainers and steppers with pedals tend to be the least accurate. Cardio machine calorie readouts are based on a formula that comes from physics, and while generally accurate, some motions are easier to standardize than others. Different users perform the exercise a little differently, and as you get better (more efficient) at a certain exercise the number of calories you burn during that activity decreases, which the machine will not pick up on. If the machine allows you to enter your body weight, the readout will be more accurate, as calorie burn is determined by effort level and work performed but also by the bodyweight of the exerciser. Gym machines get a ton of use, and if they are not calibrated from time to time the calorie readouts will be off. As long as the machine is calibrated, even if the total number of calories burned is not accurate, you can compare the number you burn from one workout session to the next and if it's higher one day than the day before, you know you did more overall work. The readouts can be used as a gauge, but if a machine says you burned 400 calories, don't assume you can go and eat 400 calories because you "burned it off." It may not necessarily be true. Furthermore, some machines include the calories your body burns just staying alive in the number, which artificially boosts the number of calories you burned off.

Is it true that exercise and a healthy diet can help reduce the chance of developing diabetes? If this is true, how can exercise and/or a good nutrition plan help prevent diabetes?

Exercise, whether aerobic or resistance-based strength training, is considered one of the most effective lifestyle habits individuals at risk to develop diabetes can adopt. In some instances, exercise has a greater beneficial effect on the management of blood sugar than changing diet or even losing weight

.

Exercise causes muscle to be more sensitive to insulin, which is the chemical signal that tells cells to absorb glucose. As a result, exercise speeds the clearance of glucose out of the blood and into muscle cells, which need glucose in higher quantities during times of increased activity. Exercise also increases circulation, thereby making more glucose available for the muscles to absorb.

Certain body fat storage and distribution patterns are red flags for health risks. Individuals who have the tendency to store fat around the midsection are often found to have other health risk factors such as high triglycerides, high blood pressure and high blood sugar levels. The portion of the abdominal fat that resides directly around the organs, known as visceral fat, as opposed to the subcutaneous portion, which is the fat just beneath the skin, is the biggest culprit for health risks. The good news is that exercise can promote abdominal fat loss preferentially over fat stored in other areas of the body.

Muscle fibers also change in response to exercise, becoming more responsive to insulin. These exercise-induced muscle fibers also have higher capillary density and greater blood supply. These changes result in lower blood sugar levels and a lowered risk of diabetes. When you are actively exercising, you will maintain increased muscle mass and along with it the associated higher metabolic demand for blood sugar at all times, including during rest. This makes diabetes less likely to develop.

Gina can be reached by visiting her website, www.homeexercisecoach.com

14. PAUL L. BARR

What are some simple things that people can do, in their day to day routine, besides working out, to see results faster?

Focus on proper nutrition. Here some simple nutritional tips that I would recommend:

1. Make sure that the 6 basic food groups are part of your daily diet:

    A. Grains

    B. Fruits

    C. Vegetables

    D. Dairy

    E. Meats

    F. Nuts

2. Start to eat more frequently throughout the day, but with smaller portions.

A person actually burns calories through eating, so it makes sense to eat more frequently.

3. Cook more of your meals at home.

Is it true that it is not a good idea to do the same exercises during each workout session? Why or Why not?

Excluding aerobic activities, such as running or biking, it depends on how often you work out per week. If you work out every day of the week, then it is NOT a good idea do the same exercises every day. The muscles you work out need approximately 48 hours to remodel. When you exercise, your muscles develop micro-tears which need time to heal and grow. If these muscles are used every day, they do not get a chance to remodel and thus do not grow stronger. If you work out every other day, or only 2-3 times a week, you are giving your muscles a chance to remodel and get bigger and stronger. The negative is that you may become bored with the same exercises every single workout.

How frequently should people change their workout routine?

It really depends on the person's goals. If a person wants to quickly lose 10 pounds of weight for a summer wedding through diet and exercise, she may not need to change routines. If a person wants to compete in the Olympics, adjustments could be made over a period of years. Workout variety is closely linked to the person's fitness goals.

After someone has reached their fitness goals, how should their workout and nutrition plan be altered if they no longer wish to lose weight or build additional muscle?

In terms of exercise there are some minimum guidelines needed to maintain fitness:

The American Heart Association suggests at least 150 minutes per week of moderate exercise or 75 minutes per week of vigorous exercise (or a combination of moderate and vigorous activity). For Example:

For moderate exercise only, if you decided to work out for 30 minutes per session, that would equate to 5 weekly sessions.

For moderate exercise only, if you decided to work out for 60 minutes per session, that would equate to 3 weekly sessions.

In terms of diet, I have provided a simple formula for estimating how many calories you need to eat per day to maintain your current weight:

Total Energy Output(TEO) = BMR + PAL + TEF

The above equation gives you a rough estimate of total calories per day

1. BMR (Men) = 1 x Body Weight(KG) x 24

   BMR(Female) = .9 x Body Weight(KG) x 24

2. PAL = BMR x Activity Level

Activity level = .10 Very little activity to .50 professional athlete

3. TEF = Total calories you eat per day x .10

Add the numbers for BMR, PAL, and TEF and this gives you an estimate of how many calories you should eat to maintain your current weight.

Remember this is an estimate only.

Is it a good idea to work out with friends or family or does that create a distraction?

Exercising in groups is a great idea, especially for people new to exercise. Group workouts can provide:

A. Motivation
B. Fun
C. Team building
D. Accountability

On the other end of the spectrum, if a person is training for the Olympic Marathon, they may alternate between solo workouts or group workouts with athletes of higher ability. In either case, working out with a friend or group can always provide a good change of pace.

Why do people have such a hard time losing belly fat?

The biggest reason is nutrition. A person could do 100 sit-ups per day for a year, but if they eat cake every day, drink beer every day, eat 1 or 2 big meals a day, they are diluting the effects of the exercise. Another reason is that they lose the belly fat too fast (no more than the 1-2 lbs. per week is suggested), or try a fad diet. They think that by not eating, the fat will disappear. To the contrary, when we deprive our body of food, we are causing our body metabolism to slow down because the body needs to conserve energy. Any food that the body does receive will be stored as fat to create a reserve because the body does not know when it will get its nutrients again. To have the best chance of losing belly fat, a person must include both proper exercise AND proper nutrition.

Is it true that it's good to have a "cheat day" where people can eat whatever they want once a week? Why is this a good or bad idea?

The simple answer is that it is perfectly acceptable to "reward" yourself for achieving a fitness and health goal. In fact, I encourage it. If a person has worked hard to lose 20-30 lbs. over a period of 6 months, they deserve to reward themselves. On the other hand, we do not want that "cheat day" to become a "cheat week" or "cheat month!"

What are the best types of exercises for getting the fastest results in the shortest period of time?

The following exercises would qualify and come under the category of interval training. The list is NOT all inclusive:

1. Circuit Training: doing a series of 5-6 exercises and then repeating the exercises.

2. Tabata: Series of exercises. Do each exercise for 4 minutes, with 20 sec of work followed by 10 sec of rest, then 20 sec work, 10 sec rest, etc. until the 4 minutes are up.

3. Boot Camps: Similar to circuit training

4. Repeats: Run 1 mile, with 1 mile recovery and then repeat X number of times

Interval training is intense training, sometimes near 90-95% of MHR (maximum heart rate). Because of the intensity, the duration of the workouts are short, under 30 minutes.

Is it true that people with diabetes have a harder time losing weight? If so, why is this the case?

In my experience, I have not detected that diabetics have a harder time losing weight than the average population.

If someone needs to quickly lose a few pounds for a special occasion, what's the best way they can do this?

There are no "quick" fixes. The best way to lose weight, safely and effectively, is through diet and exercise.

The general rule is 1-2 lbs. per week or 1% of current body weight per week.

For example, if a woman wants to lose 20 lbs. for a wedding, she would need to allocate approximately from 10 weeks or 2 months to 20 weeks or 5 months.

If a quick loss diet sounds too good to be true, it is!

Does a person have to check with their doctor before beginning a workout program with a personal trainer?

In my practice, I follow this procedure:

A. Have the client fill out a complete health history form. If the client has any current medical issues with heart, diabetes, etc., I automatically have them get a doctors permission before working with the client. If the client has no known issues, I check their information against the CAD (Coronary Artery Disease) risk factors, and then determine if they need a doctors permission

What type of shoes should people wear when working out?

Some type of quality athletic shoe is fine: cross train shoe, running shoe. No department store sneakers, please!

In addition to working out, what are some of the most beneficial activities to participate in and why are these activities so beneficial/healthy?

In general, any type of group activity is highly recommended. If you are a runner or biker, for example, there are hundreds of great clubs around the country. Participating in a group with common interests, provides friendship and fun. Participating in a club can help push you to get better at your particular sport.

Why do people say breakfast is the most important meal of the day? Is there any truth to this?

Think of it this way: if you started your car and left it running for 7-8 hours, do you think it would need gas? The answer: of course.

Now, a human sleeps for 7-8 hours, is its body still working, keeping your heart pumping and lungs breathing? Yes. Do you think after not eating for 7-8 hours that the body might want some food? Absolutely. That is why breakfast is the most important meal of the day. If you skip breakfast, you will become listless and tired. Consider breakfast as your fuel fill up for the day.

What are the best foods people should eat to gain energy and why are these foods important?

The best foods for energy contain carbohydrates. Carbs are the body's primary energy source. Some great foods containing carbs are:

Bananas: because they are easy to eat and digest and are loaded with fast-acting carbohydrates (one large banana provides 31 grams of carbs), bananas make the perfect pre-exercise or post-exercise snack. Just be sure to have your banana with some form of protein after exercise to promote muscle recovery and repair.

Berries: strawberries, blueberries, and other berries are among the most nutritious sources of carbohydrate. They are rich in vitamins, minerals, and phytonutrients that promote health and performance in all kinds of ways. Berries are not the most concentrated source of carbs, however (a full cup of strawberries contains just 12 grams), so don't rely on them too heavily to meet your daily carbohydrate needs.

Brown Rice: cereal grains such as brown rice are among the richest sources of carbohydrate. One cup of brown rice has 45 grams of carbohydrate. Whole grains such as brown rice are considered healthier than refined grains such as white rice because they contain more fiber, vitamins, and minerals. They are also absorbed more slowly (i.e., their glycemic index is lower), so they provide more lasting energy and promote less fat storage.

Whole-wheat pasta: is also high in carbs. One cup of whole-wheat spaghetti provides 37 grams. As with other grain-based foods, whole-grain pasta supplies more nutrition, yields longer-lasting energy, and promotes less fat storage than regular pasta. Serve it with a protein, such as shellfish or meatballs made with lean ground beef or turkey, and you get a lower glycemic index meal for even longer-lasting energy.

Paul can be reached at
Never Give Up Fitness
www.nevergiveupfitness.com
Twitter: @PaulLBarr
Facebook: http://www.facebook.com/NeverGiveUpFitness

CONCLUSION

Congratulations on making it to the end of this book! We hope that you realize and appreciate the immense level of real world knowledge that you've just acquired. The one thing you may be feeling at this point is a bit of "information overload" due to the many tips, pieces of advice, and strategies that are jammed into this book. If you are feeling overwhelmed about everything you've just learned, allow us to offer you one final piece of advice: take a day to let your brain absorb all of the information you just learned. As they say: "Sleep on it". If you attempt to try and remember and implement everything you just learned, your efforts may tend to be scattered and a bit unorganized. Instead, take a day off from the information. If you do this, you're likely to find that you develop a sense of clarity and a better perspective on the information.

Once you've taken a day to allow yourself to re-focus in this way, we encourage you to slowly go back through the book, highlighting and writing down the actionable information that you intend to implement. Simply reading and understanding the information is not enough. By writing down the information that you plan on implementing, it will allow you to put a clear plan of action into place for yourself.

As you go through the information, don't worry about the order in which you write things down. The first thing to do is to just get the information down on paper. There are many great strategies and tips within this book, but the goal here is for you to extract the exact advice that you will be taking action on. Don't worry if you are unsure about whether or not you will be taking immediate action on certain ideas. Just write down everything that you may possibly take action on.

Once you've compiled this list of action steps and possible action steps, begin to prioritize this list. In other words, re-write the list with the actions that you know you're going to take at the top of the list and the action items that you are least likely to do towards the bottom of the list. By organizing your list in this way, you will be able to build a practical, useable to-do list from the information you learned in this book. Once you've done this, you will be in an excellent position to start taking focused steps with clarity and purpose.

As we mentioned at the beginning of this book, most peddlers of fitness products and information hope that you keep buying their stuff. In keeping with the rebellious nature of this book, we encourage you to stop buying more fitness stuff and start implementing what you just learned within these pages! Just as we have shared interviews with real-world experts who actually do what they talk about in this book, it is our hope that you, as the reader, will take real-world action on the information you've found here.

Here's wishing you all the best in your action-taking fitness and nutrition endeavors!

Sincerely,

Andy Adami

SouthPeakPress.com